An Easy Way
To Understand
Aromatherapy
&
Essential Oils

Also By Brian B Jacques

His very popular Series of Mini-Health Books includes:

- An Easy Way To Understand Eczema and Psoriasis
- An Easy Way To Understand Stress and Depression
- Amino Acids & Enzymes—What Are They & Why Do You Need Them
- An Easy Way To Understand Vitamins and Minerals
- An Easy Way To Understand Crohn's Disease and IBD
- An Easy Way To Understand Body Building For Men And Women
- An Easy Way To Understand Parasites, Worms, Candida, Constipation & Detoxing
- An Easy Way To Understand Alzheimer's Disease
- An Easy Way To Understand Herpes
- An Easy Way To Understand Parkinson's Disease
- An Easy Way To Understand Autism
- An Easy Way To Understand Fibromyalgia
- The Little A–Z Dictionary of Herbal Remedies
- Effective Methods To Stop Smoking
- The Magic Of Vitamins & Minerals
- An Easy Way To Understand Your Body Systems
- An Easy Way To Understand Erectile Dysfunction
- An Easy Way To Understand Heart Disease, High Blood Pressure & Stroke
- An Easy Way To Understand Detoxing For Men & Women
- How To Lose Weight After 40
- How To Lose Weight And Maintain Your Ideal Weight Permanently
- Herbs For Healing—101 Herbal Remedies—What Are They, What Are They Used For
- Eat Wholefoods And Take Supplements

All these books are also available as Kindle Editions (available from the Kindle Store on Amazon.com, and other countries Amazon sites where the Kindle platform is supported.) Many of these books are also available for the Barnes and Noble "Nook". In addition, all these titles will shortly be available as print editions from the Amazon website.

An Easy Way
To Understand
Aromatherapy
&
Essential Oils

Brian B Jacques.

Part of a Series of Mini Health Books

Wisdom For Life Media

4   Brian B Jacques.

Publisher: Wisdom For Life Media

While they have made every effort to verify the information provided in this book, neither the author nor the publisher assumes any responsibility for errors in, omissions from, or different interpretation of the subject matter.

The information herein may be subject to varying laws, regulations, and practices in different areas, states and countries. The purchaser or reader assumes all responsibility for use of the information.

All information included within this book is for educational purposes only. The author and publishers do not attempt to diagnose or treat any medical conditions, be it to do with health, diet or exercise.

If you consider that you may have or already have any kind of medical condition, then, you should consult a qualified medical practitioner or doctor before starting any aromatherapy or essential oil program or treatment suggested in this book.

This book is not intended for anyone under the age of 18 years, nor is it intended for breast feeding or pregnant women, underweight people or anyone with eating disorders or a health condition that requires special diets or medical treatment.

The author and publishers disclaim any liability for any loss however caused by anyone using the information contained in this book.

Images

All images are either copyright the author or are used under the terms of a royalty free license.

ISBN - 13: 978-1516951413

ISBN - 10: 1516951417

Printed and published in the United States of America

"Education is the kindling of a flame, not the filling of a vessel."—Socrates

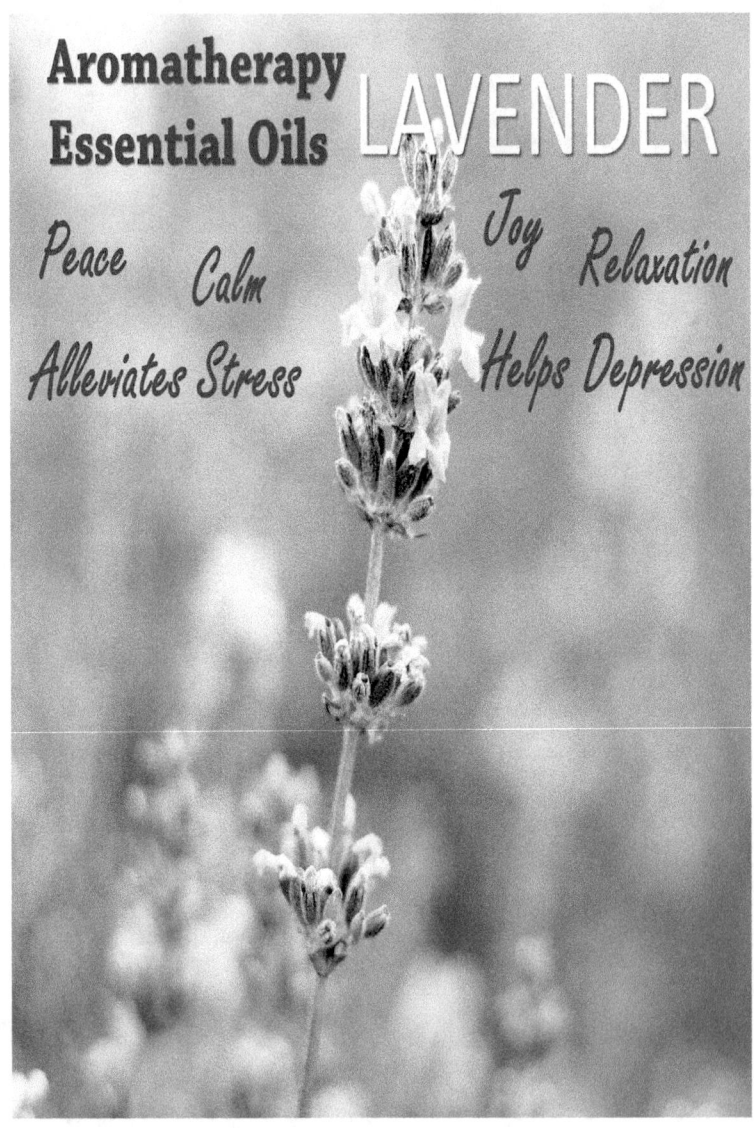

Contents

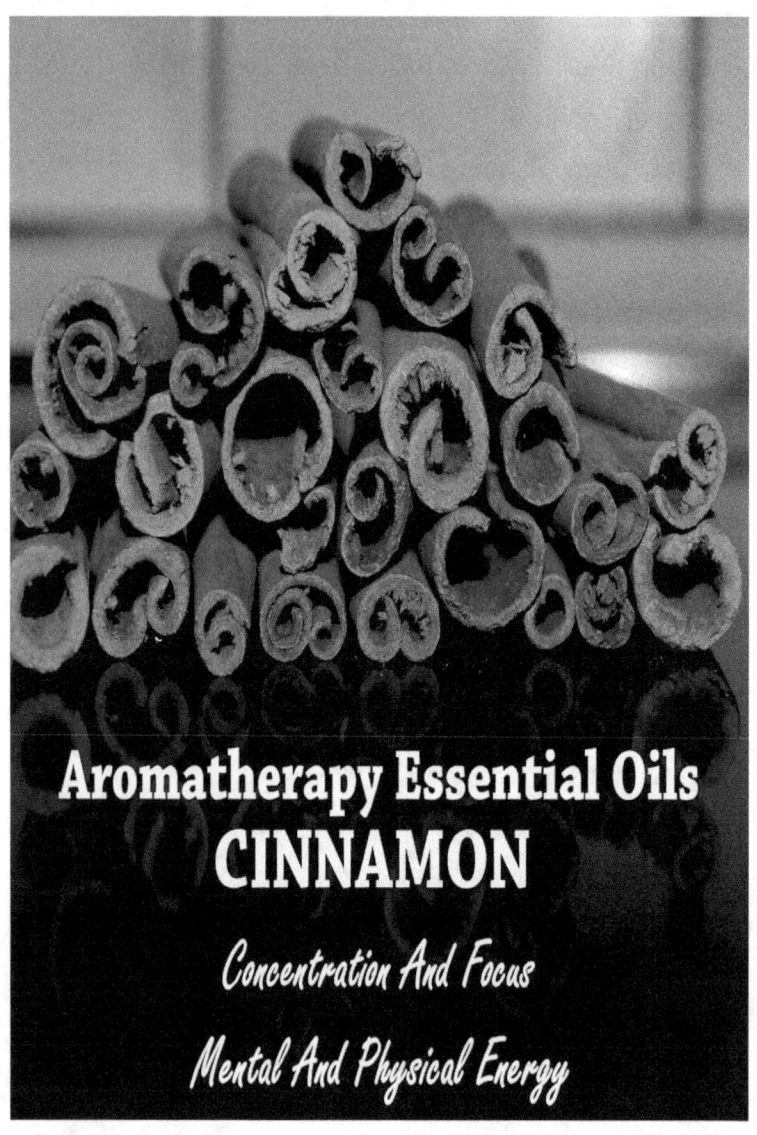

Acknowledgment

To the many people I have come into contact with throughout my life, whose belief in me has made everything possible and worthwhile.

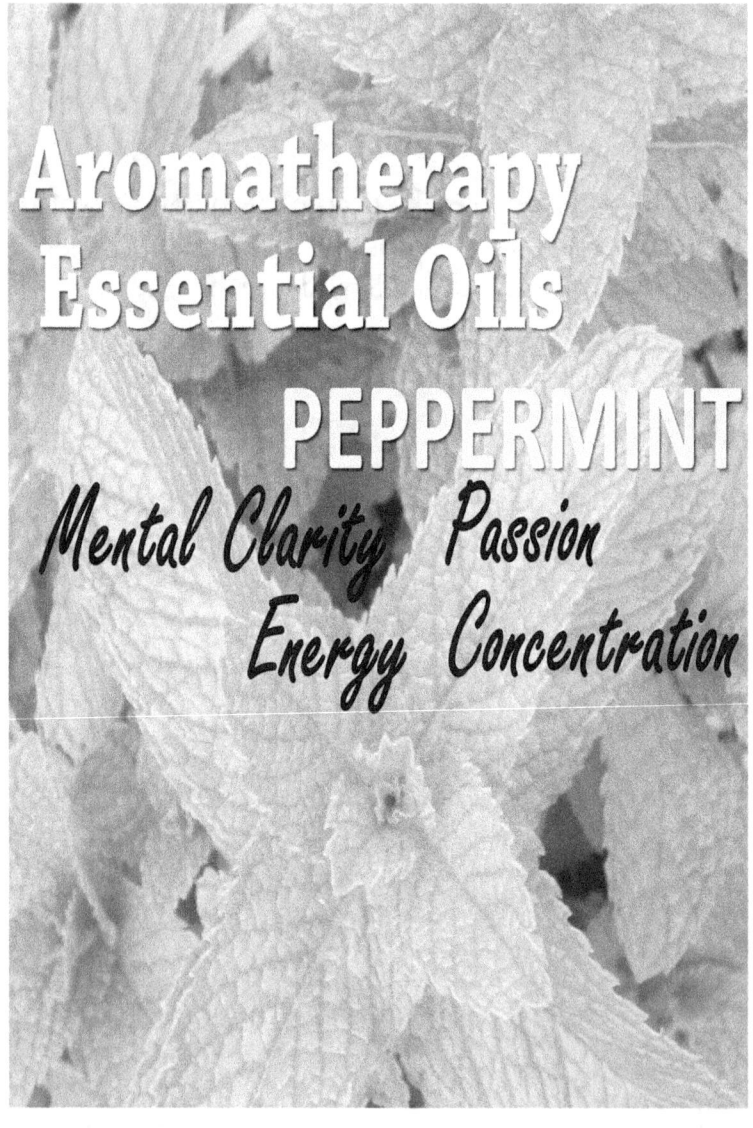

Introduction

Did you know that there are over 100 references to essential oils in the Bible? Perhaps the best known reference is that of the birth of the baby Jesus, when gold frankincense and myrrh were brought to him as gifts.

At that time these valuable herbs, oils and spices were transported vast distances across hot deserts by Arab merchants to satisfy an ever increasing demand. The two most sought after items were frankincense and myrrh. And because demand outstripped supply, they were valued at a far higher price than gems or precious metals.

In fact the origins of aromatherapy can be traced back over 3,000 years—long before the birth of Christ. Perhaps the Egyptians can claim a lot of the credit for the birth of the use of essential oils. The Egyptians loved to use fragrances—and they would do so at every possible opportunity. They would use fragrances after bathing to help keep their skin soft and to exude a fragrance as well.

Through the centuries the Egyptians continued to enhance their use of essential oils for use in cosmetics, incense, medicines and perfumes. In addition, the Egyptians developed a real expertise in the use of essential oils for use in the mummification process of their royalty as they prepared them for their journey into the afterlife.

Not to be outdone, the Greeks and Romans played an important part too. The Greeks enjoyed using aromatic plants, and they laid mint leaves on the floors of their temples. The Romans placed laurels of bay, mint and rosemary on their head to celebrate important occasions and battle victories. They were also well known for their use of lavender to scent their bath water.

Hippocrates (460-370BC) who is considered the father of medicine was a great believer in scented massages and aromatic baths as well as the internal use of various herbs. He believed that there was a natural way to treat disease by using patient observation to determine what symptoms were present.

The term "aromatherapy" was first used by French scientist Rene-Maurice Gattefosse (1881-1950), while conducting research into the antiseptic, cosmetic and healing properties of essential oils; he severely burned his hand when there was an explosion in his laboratory. He immediately plunged his hand into a vat of pure lavender oil. The result, the swelling immediately subsided, the wound healed quickly and there was no scarring afterwards.

Another important figure was a French doctor Jean Valnet (1920-1995) who earned the accolade of being the "father of modern phy-to-aromatherapy". He used essential oils in World War 11 to treat battle wounds when there was a shortage of medicines.

The art of aromatherapy has a rich heritage, and it can play an important part as an alternative or complementary medicinal treatment for a variety of modern day illnesses, as well as being a great way to bring harmony and tranquility into everyday life.

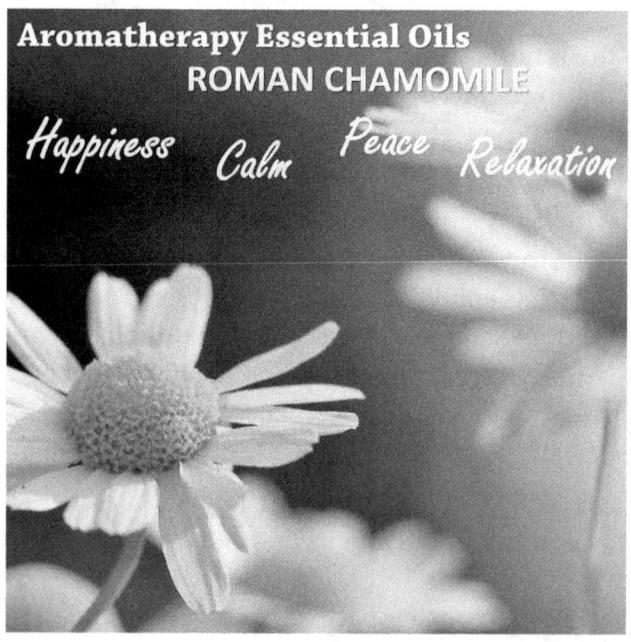

1. Understanding The Art of Aromatherapy

Aromatherapy involves the use of plant parts (leaves, fruits, flowers, seeds, wood, bark, berries resin, and roots) and the oils extracted from them to assist in altering the mood, mental, emotional and physical health of humans. If you are just beginning to learn the secrets of aromatherapy and essential oils then this is a great book for you to read. You'll learn the basics of aromatherapy and the power that plants have to heal humans.

The majority of oils are extracted using a steam distillation process and some are captured using a solvent such as alcohol. The structure of essential oils allows them to be mixed with other oils and creams or they can be used in a variety of ways to affect your emotional, physical and cellular needs.

There are a few important points to bear in mind when working with essential oils:

- Only use 100% authentic pure essential oils—do not use synthetic essential oils.

- If a recipe says 2 drops, and you think 4 drops will make the blend twice as effective, think again. The difference in reaction between 2 drops and 4 drops could be somewhere in the stratosphere—in other words, don't do it!

- Understand about each individual's allergies and skin sensitivity—what may work well and be suitable for one person may cause discomfort for another person

- Apart from lavender and tea tree (but not for everyone) do not use neat essential oils, always use a carrier oil.

- Bergamot, lemon, lime and bitter orange are photo-sensitizing which means that a person should avoid going out in sunlight for at least 12 hours after using these oils on the skin.

- In case of skin sensitivity or irritation use vegetable oil to purge the oil from the skin.

- Keep all essential oils out of the reach of children and pets. Remember essential oils are very concentrated and can cause serious harm if swallowed by a child, a pet as well as an adult.

- Store all essential oils in dark amber or dark blue colored bottles and away from light and heat.

- Avoid oils that are sold in clear glass bottles. Light will destroy the effectiveness of the oil.

- Do not use plastic bottles. Essential oils can degrade the plastic.

- Essential oils can strain clothing and it will be very difficult to get the stain out. Also, essential oils can damage the finish on furniture, which like stains on cloths; can be very difficult to remove.

The way that aromatherapy works is by absorbing the oil into the skin, or inhaling it through the nose. Some essential oils can be ingested, but this should only be done under the supervision of a qualified aromatherapist and also tell your doctor that you are using essential oils.

You can put diluted essential oils on various parts of the body such as the crown of your head, behind the ears, upper and lower back, abdomen, temples, neck, under the nose, inside the wrists, and on the collarbone. All these areas are considered pulse points. These are basically warmer parts of the body which work as a natural diffuser to disperse the oils into the air so that you can inhale them.

Using the correct essential oils can assist with many parts of your life in addition to improving your environment too. As an example, to create calming ambiance in your home, diffuse some lavender in the family room. If you want to wake up fresher in the morning then add some lemon oil and mint to your bath wash. Have a headache? Then soak a compress in some eucalyptus and place it on your forehead or neck. And what about morning sickness? Try smelling some lemon essential oil and it will disappear. All these examples work—you just have to try them.

The reason essential oils work this way is that they are lipophilic, meaning they dissolve in lipids or fats. In simple terms, essential oils can cross the membrane of a body cell. This means that essential oils can affect the body cells in very healing ways. Most people have heard of antibiotics, but antibiotics do not cross the cell membrane; therefore you can begin to understand how the use of essential oils may be able to help you have a healthier body.

2. Benefits of Smells for Healing

We are constantly inhaling smells. It is something we do automatically. When you are in the countryside and go outside first thing in the morning and breathe in the fresh air, you get the scent of trees, grass and flowers. If you are in a city you may breathe in traffic fumes and the often unpleasant smell that entails. Some smells have a good association for us and some possibly not so good. Smells remind us of things. Lavender may remind you of opening a drawer containing linen and the beautiful smell that is released. The smell of fresh lemon reminds you of a close friend. Smells involve all aspects of our lives from improving memory to affecting our mood.

Recent research suggests that our skin can "smell" different scents which can have a healing effect on the body. In this case you may or may not be aware of the scent but there is a health benefit there for you.

Various research has been done using brain scans to see what effect smelling essential oils has on the brain. The hypothalamus—the center for hormones which control drive and energy—springs to life. The conclusion: smells can make you feel more centered and energetic.

Different smells create different responses. For example: mint is more energizing, lavender is more calming. Various scents can be chosen for different body requirements. In addition, scents can be combined to make a specific treatment for particular body conditions.

- **Improve Energy** – Feeling tired and lethargic? You can use essential oils to help energize yourself. Many smells can help you feel more energized, such as citrus and mint.

- **Relieve Stress** – Everyone has a degree of stress in their lives, but with the right essential oils you can reduce your stress levels. Consider lemon oil, lavender and peppermint. All these can be helpful for lowering stress levels.

- **Reduce Anger** – Certain stress responses can cause angry outbursts. If this is you, then why not try using lemon oil as a stress reliever.

- **Memory Enhancement** – Sage and orange are good essential oils for memory enhancement. One way to trigger memory is to smell the same things you smelled at the first time you experienced the memory.

- **Natural Antidepressant** -- Do you suffer from depression or experience sadness on occasions? Essential oils can help. Chamomile, jasmine, lavender and peppermint are good scents to help reduce depressive tendencies.

- **Get Rid of a Headache** – Eucalyptus, peppermint, rosemary and sandalwood are all good scents to help eliminate a headache. If you get persistent headaches then the best thing to do is determine the cause and treat that. For example, if you are stressed out, you can use lavender instead of one of the above.

- **Better Sleep** – One of the most important factors in maintaining good health aside from eating a balanced wholefood diet, taking natural vitamin and mineral supplements and exercising is getting adequate and restful sleep. Any of the calming scents will help you such as lavender and chamomile plus many others.

- **Pain Reduction**– Essential oils can be a great help for dealing with chronic pain. The oil can be incorporated into a compress and applied to the affected area; the oil can also be inhaled to help your body relax.

Combining aromatherapy with traditional medicine can prove very beneficial. Consult a trained aromatherapist as well as your doctor. When used correctly aromatherapy is safe and effective for all types of issues.

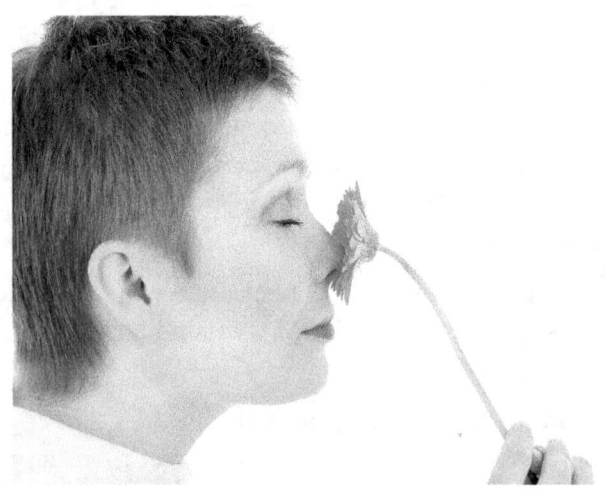

3 Essential Oils And Safety Issues

Many people are of the opinion that there is no harm in using essential oils. However, studies have shown that excessive use of essential oils can be harmful for proper lung function; in addition the oils can become less effective. It is therefore important to remember that even natural ingredients when used to excess can cause unwanted side effects.

- **Proper Dilution** – Essential oils are highly concentrated, and if used undiluted on the skin they could burn you. I am sure you have heard the phrase "less is more" this is especially important when using essential oils.

- **Take care when using Citrus** – photosensitizing molecules are involved here, therefore if any citrus oils are applied to the skin it is important that you are not exposed to direct sunlight for at least 12 hours otherwise you could receive a burn.

- **Check the Labeling** – Essential oils are required to have the name of the oil and the country of origin on the label. Make sure it does.

- **Store as if they are Medicines** – Essential oils should be stored in a cool dark place to ensure they maintain their effectiveness and freshness. In addition, make sure that any essential oils are stored away from where children and pets can reach them. Remember, essential oils can cause major health issues if they are used incorrectly, in much the same way as medicines can.

- **Research First**– Understand what an essential oil is appropriate for before using it—especially if it is one that you have not used before. A qualified aromatherapist will be able to advise you if you are unsure.

- **Don't Ingest Essential Oils**– Essential oils should not be ingested unless under the supervision of a trained aromatherapist or physician.

- **Avoid the Eye Area** – Don't put essential oils near the eyes or other mucus membranes.

- **Keep Away from Flames** – Avoid putting essential oils near a flame as some of them are flammable and can explode. If you intend using essential oils with a candle, then pour the oil into the molten wax, not on to the flame.

- **Only Inhale for a Maximum of One Hour** – Only inhale vapors from essential oils for a total of an hour or less each day. Several seconds are all that are really needed. Some respiratory issues have occurred from overuse.

Remember essential oils are safe and effective when used in the correct way and in moderation. Take time to learn about the methods that are used and which oils are recommended for specific health issues before trying them yourself.

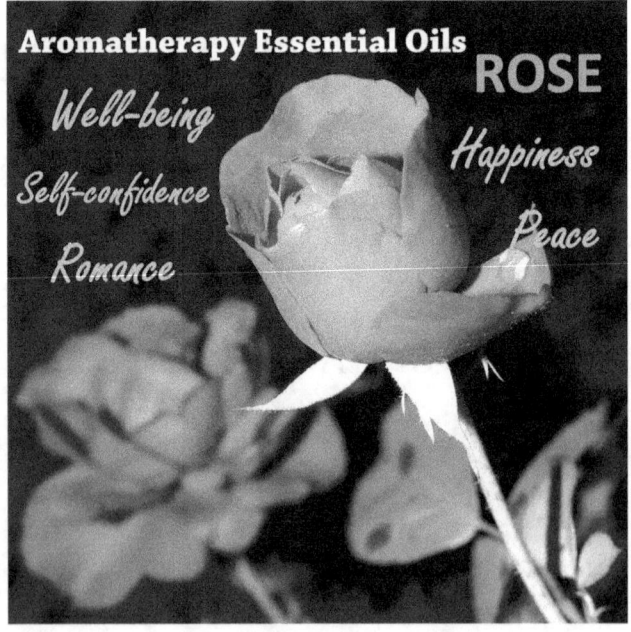

4 Storing Essential Oils

Correct storage of essential oils is important to ensure a long shelf life—that the oils do not lose their effectiveness—and one way to do this is to store them in a cool dark place.

- **Dark Colored Glass Bottles**: Excluding ultra violet light is the key issue here. This is why the majority of essential oils are stored in dark amber colored glass bottles. Other colors are sometimes used such as blue. The important part is that the glass is resistant to ultra-violent light.

- **Dark Place**: Even with the special dark colored glass it is still important to put the bottles in a dark place. Instead of leaving them out, place them inside a cabinet.

- **Cool Place**: The color of the glass and placing the bottles in a dark place is only one part of correct storage. The final part is placing the bottles in a cool environment to prolong effectiveness and shelf life.

  If you do not have air conditioning in your home, then place the bottles— especially citrus essential oils, in a refrigerator. Certain oils may solidify, if this happens, remove them from the refrigerator say half an hour before use to let them warm up.

- **Store Out of Reach**: Make sure you store your essential oils out of reach of pets and children. Essential oils can be harmful if ingested or can burn the skin if they are undiluted. Treat them like you would medicines.

And finally, do not use plastic bottles with essential oils in high concentrations. A few drops of essential oil that has been diluted in a carrier oil may be safe in a plastic container, but it is not recommended. Undiluted essential oils have the ability to degrade plastic containers which can result in them decomposing.

5 What Equipment Do You Need to Get Started

If you decide to try aromatherapy and use essential oils, then you will need some basic equipment. The equipment you will need will depend on what you decide to use the oils for. The following is a list of the different types.

Oil Burners

Many different types of oil burners are available at various price points from electric, ceramic, glass, metal, and soapstone. Oil burners fill the room with the scent of the oil you have put into them.

Whatever type of oil burner you choose, they all work on a similar principle—they warm the oil which then causes it to evaporate into the air. The electric ones plug into a wall socket while the others use a tea-light candle.

Warming essential oils can reduce some of the medicinal benefits, but on the flip-side, it can create a great ambiance in a room, and get the oil quickly into the air.

One of the great advantages of an oil burner is that you can mix many different oils together to create your own "scents" and treatment regimes.

Compresses

A compress can be hot or cold and made from gauze, wash clothes or essential oil sheets. Put a few drops of oil into water then soak the compress in the mixture, wring the compress out and apply to the affected area.

As an example, for a headache, you can place the compress on your forehead or neck; for a sprain, place the compress on the affected area. Essential oils can be ingested through the skin or inhaled through the nose.

Glass Bottles

Purchase some amber or dark blue colored bottles that exclude ultra violet light so that you can mix your own medicinal oil treatments. As an example, mix mint and lemon into a bottle for an energy boost; chamomile and lavender into another for a calming effect. There are many different oil recipes that you can mix, some suggestions are described elsewhere in this book.

If you intend to rub oils onto your skin, then you need to mix them with a carrier oil such as coconut oil, jojoba oil or sweet almond oil. Essential oils on their own can be very strong and can cause skin burns if they are not diluted in a carrier oil.

You will find it useful having a selection of bottles available so that you can premix your oils ready for use.

Diffusers

Diffusers are designed to distribute the essential oils into the air so that they can be inhaled through the nose and then processed by the body. There are pluses and minuses for each one. Choose the one that is most suitable for your requirements.

There are several different types of diffusers that you can use:

- **Evaporative** – Uses a fan which blows air onto a cloth or pad which contains drops of essential oils to evaporate the oil into the air which is then dispersed around the room. It makes a room smell good and fresh. However, it loses some of the health benefits of the essential oils by destroying them in the evaporation process.

- **Nebulizing** – This works on the same principle as a perfume atomizer. It converts the oil into a fine mist with a burst of air. This process helps conserve the oil and avoids wastage.

- **Humidifying** – This process uses a combination of vibration and air to convert the essential oils into small particles that are perfect for inhalation. This process works great for respiratory problems and for infusing an entire room with essential oils.

- **Ultrasonic** – This method of distribution uses vibrations to convert the essential oil into a very fine mist which creates tiny micro particles that are easily absorbed into the lungs. It's accomplishes this without the use of any type of heat.

- **Heat** – This method uses a flame or electrical connection to heat the essential oil and cause it to evaporate into the air. Many oils are degraded with the use of heat and this can destroy the medicinal benefit.

The type of diffuser you use will depend on what you intend to use it for and your budget. Diffusion is very versatile. You can improve your home environment, reduce stress levels, help with insomnia, feel happier, be more alert, have more energy, get great health benefits and even reduce airborne pathogens which are harmful to the body when they are breathed in.

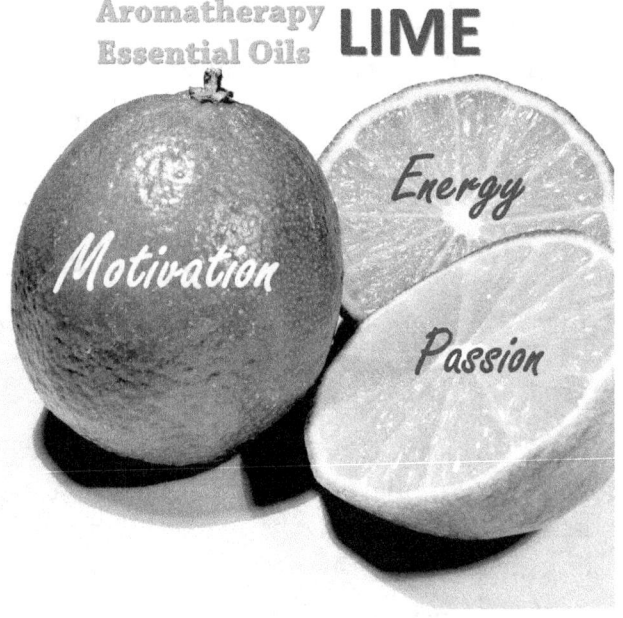

6. Plant Parts Used And Extraction Processes

Why the name "Essential" oils? It's all to do with science and the word quintessence which means an "extract of a substance". How this works is still difficult to describe, but it is linked to dynamic forces that are associated with the universe. Essential oils are classified as an oil because they are insoluble in water, but become soluble in oils such as sunflower oil, sweet almond oil.

Elsewhere in this book I caution you to follow stated drops of an essential oil in a recipe this is because essential oils are at a minimum 50 times more potent than the plant they are extracted from.

There are several hundred thousand plants in the world, but relatively few of these are suitable for extracting essential oils. Some plants contain such small quantities of oil that it is not cost effective to use them.

Depending on the plant, essential oils can be extracted from the flowers, stem, root, bark, seeds or resin. You may find the following table useful to see which plant parts are used to extract oils.

Plant Parts	Essential Oils
Flowers	Chamomile – Roman, Clove, Helichrysum, Jasmine, Lavender, Neroli (Orange Blossom), Rose, Thyme, Ylang Ylang
Leaves	Cinnamon, Clary Sage, Eucalyptus, Geranium, Lavender, Lemongrass, Marjoram, Oregano, Patchouli, Peppermint, Rosemary, Tea Tree, Thyme
Bark	Cinnamon
Roots	Ginger
Needles	Cypress, Pine
Fruit peel	Bergamot, Grapefruit, Pink, Lemon, Lime, Sweet Orange, Tangerine, Mandarin
Resin	Frankincense, Myrrh
Heartwood	Sandalwood

Extraction Processes

Various extraction processes can be used to extract the oils from the plant. The most common ones are: steam distillation, cold pressing and alcohol extraction.

Steam Distillation

In this process the plant is placed into a closed container and steam is added which passes through the plant. Heat from the steam assists in opening parts of the plant that contain the oils. Once the oils are released they rise to the top along with the steam. The top part of the container contains a cooling system in which cold water is added to cool the steam. As the cooling takes place, the oil and water separate. It is then a simple matter to skin the oil off the top of the water. These are then the essential oils that are used in aromatherapy.

Cold Pressed

A cold pressed system is used to extract oils from citrus fruits as well as nuts and seeds. In this process no heat is used. The oils are forced out under mechanical pressure along with a certain amount of water, which will evaporate, leaving just the oils behind.

Alcohol Extraction

And no, I am not talking about the alcohol that you drink. This alcohol is formed from a different molecular structure and is used for plants which cannot tolerate heat. The alcohol opens the plant to release the oils then with further alcohol distillation the oils are finally extracted.

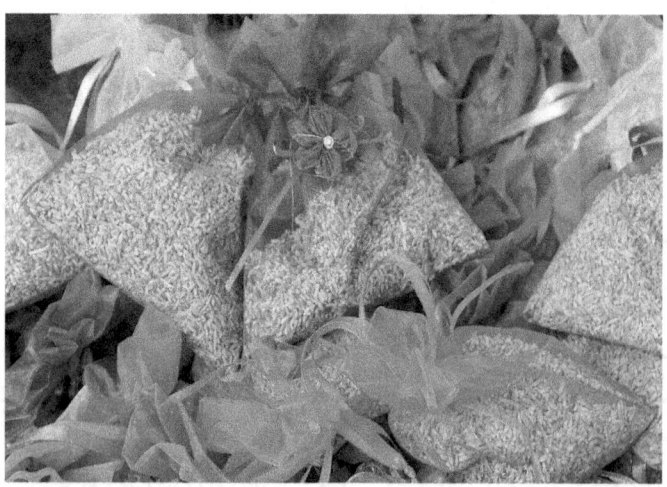

7. Essential Oil Families

To make life easier, essential oils are grouped into "families" as follows: Citrus, Floral, Herbaceous, Spice, Wood and Resin and Camphorous. See the descriptions below.

Citrus

- **Bergamot**. *Rejuvenating and Supportive.* Bergamot has a sweet aroma smelling of citrus. Used to ease anxiety and tension and stress.

- **Lemon**. *Clean and Crisp.* The clean and crisp scent of lemon is great for cleansing the body and home.

- **Grapefruit – Pink**. *Energy and Elevating.* Pink grapefruit is well known for lifting the spirits and dispelling gloom.

- Mandarin – Red. *Tranquility and Calming.* Red Mandarin has a sweet, tangy aroma which promotes a feeling of calmness.

Floral

- **Helichrysum**. *Restoring and Recuperate.* Helichrysum has a strong scent and is often used to treat skin injuries.

- **Chamomile – Roman**. *Comforting and Subtle.* This versatile oil is used for many different health conditions.

- **Rose**. *Contentment and Fondness.* Used for centuries in perfumes, Rose exudes a sweet deep scent that can also be used for various health conditions.

- **Jasmine**. *Romance and Tranquility.* Used for centuries to enhance sexual feelings. Jasmine exudes a very intense aroma.

- **Neroli**. *Influential and Appealing.* Neroli projects a sweet floral aroma which provides support for the nervous, digestive and intestinal systems.

- **Ylang Ylang**. *Equilibrium and Yearning.* Ylang Ylang Provides an enriching and sensual experience through its exotic floral ambiance.

Herbaceous

- **Clary Sage**. *Stress and Uplifting.* Clary Sage has a clear, herbal aroma that eases stress during monthly menstrual cycles as well as during menopause.

- **Geranium.** *Nurtures and Reinforces.* Geranium is often used for treating skin conditions and menstrual issues.
- **Lavender.** *Soothing and Radiant.* Lavender with its unique aroma has long been prized for its multitude of uses.
- **Lemon Grass.** *Refreshing and Soothing.* Lemon Grass provides a revitalizing element especially for the respiratory and nervous systems.
- **Marjoram.** *Calming and Reinforcing.* Marjoram's spicy scent helps ease tension and calms nerves.
- **Oregano.** *Cleansing and Protecting.* Oregano has a powerful scent which is often used for respiratory system problems and digestive system support.
- **Pine.** *Rejuvenate and Invigorate.* An uplifting experience is felt by inhaling the smell of pine.
- **Thyme.** *Invigorating and Restoring.* Thyme's warm scent provides support for the nervous system.

Camphorous

- **Eucalyptus.** *Cool and Refreshing.* The aroma of Eucalyptus has a calming effect and supports the immune system.
- **Peppermint.** *Crisp and Energetic.* Peppermint projects a strong mint aroma which is used for various health conditions.
- **Rosemary.** *Distinct and Current.* Rosemary exudes a camphorous scent which is stimulating for the mind and body.
- **Tea Tree.** *Reinstate and Endure.* Tea Tree possesses a fresh, warm camphorous aroma which is used for various types of infections.

Spice

- **Cinnamon.** *Subtle and Comforting.* Projects a feeling of warmth. Stimulates the soul with its spicy aroma.
- **Clove.** *Release and Bolster.* Clove provides excellent pain relief and exudes a spicy, rich scent.

Wood and Resin

- **Frankincense.** *Focus and Uplifting.* Calming and uplifting, Frankincense projects a woody, spicy scent.

- **Myrrh.** *Flexible and Strong.* Myrrh exudes a spicy aroma which has been used in religious ceremonies since ancient times. It also projects endurance and strength.

- **Patchouli.** *Equilibrium and Supporting.* Patchouli has an earthy scent and is well known for treating skin conditions.

- **Sandalwood.** *Regularize and Inspire.* A true luxury oil, Sandalwood provides a calming effective during times of anxiety and stress.

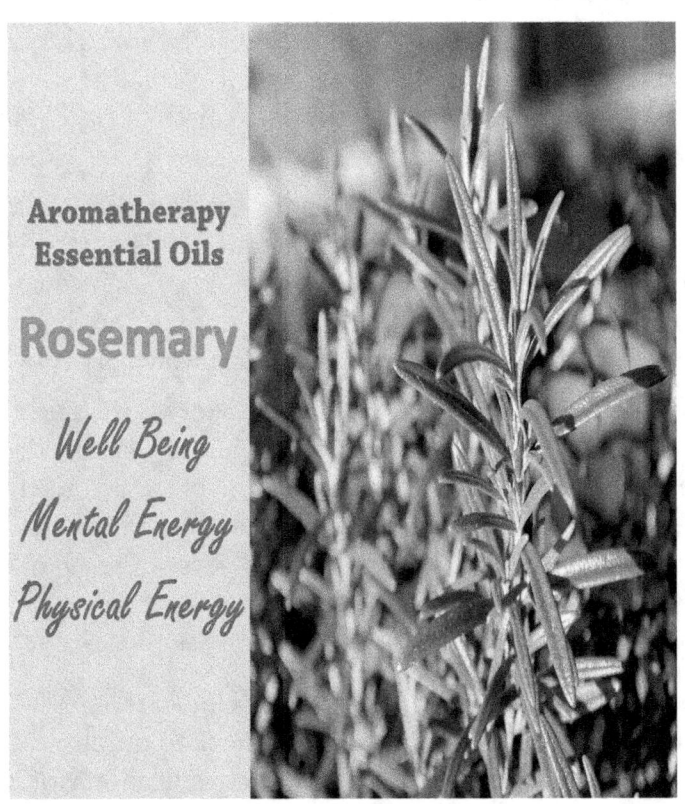

8. Blending Essential Oils

After you have used single essential oils, the next stage is you will probably want to mix different oils together. We call this blending. When you blend two or more essential oils together you can create some really exquisite fragrances—which you can never get with just a single oil.

Following a few basic rules will make for a better blend—and result for you. When you blend oils together, it is a good idea to have paper and pencil handy so that you can write the formula down that you have created, in case you want to mix it again. If you don't do this, then, it may prove difficult to recreate the same fragrance in the future.

Consider what you intend to use the oil blend for? Then consider the chemical properties of the essential oils. What is the thickness (viscosity) of the oil? And what about the volatility (is it reactive) of the oil?

Complementary oils should be blended together. It is not advisable to blend a calming oil with one that is energizing, if your goal is to create a calming blend—it will defeat the purpose of what you are trying to accomplish. Therefore it is important to understand the properties of the various oils you intend to blend before you start.

Always work methodically. Prepare labels for your blends. Include the essential oils you have put in the blend and how many drops. Put the date the blend was created, and what the blend is for. Always put your blends in dark amber or dark blue bottles, and preferable in a dark cool place. And keep your essential oils out of reach of children and pets.

"Notes"

Before we get into blending, we will take a look at "notes". There are many different types of essential oils available to purchase. To make life easy they have been placed into three classifications for blending purposes. These classifications are called "notes", and they are centered on the essential oils chemical properties.

The three classifications are called top notes, middle notes and base notes. Top notes are the most powerful as well as being volatile. They are absorbed quickly into the skin and evaporate quickly after about 30 minutes or so.

Top notes tend to be light, stimulating and uplifting.

Middle notes comprise the majority of essential oils. They tend to be more stable. Many of them do not have a strong scent which tends to release over a period from one minute to three hours. Essential oils in this classification tend to be soothing and balancing to the body as well as giving balance and stability to a blend.

Base notes are less volatile they often have a heavy scent and evaporate slowly. These essential oils tend to hold the fragrance in the blend longer, as opposed to blends without a base note, where the fragrance tends to degrade more quickly.

You may find the following chart useful to help you determine which essential oil belongs in which "note".

Top Notes	Middle Notes	Base Notes
Bergamot	Chamomile	Frankincense
Eucalyptus	Cinnamon	Ginger
Grapefruit	Clary Sage	Helichrysum
Lavender	Clove	Myrrh
Lemon	Geranium	Patchouli
Lemongrass	Jasmine	Sandalwood
Mandarin	Marjoram	
Orange	Neroli	
Peppermint	Pine	
Tea Tree	Rose	
	Rosemary	
	Thyme	
	Ylang Ylang	

There are two main types of blends: aromatic and therapeutic. An aromatic blend is something that is going to smell great and give pleasure. A therapeutic blend is something that is going to give relief to a health condition. Having said that, the fragrance of a therapeutic blend needs to be taken into consideration. If the scent is not good, then chances are there may be a resistance to using it.

As you start blending oils together, it might be a good idea to limit the number to three or four at the most. If you start blending more, it might be overwhelming until you have gained more blending experience. As a general rule, oils from the same family will blend well together. Here is a useful guide.

Top Notes	3 Drops
Middle Notes	2 Drops
Base Notes	1 Drop

The 3, 2, 1 rule is a good one to follow when you are starting out blending essential oils.

Take contraindications into account when formulating blends. As an example, certain oils should not be used during pregnancy. So, if you are creating a blend for someone who is pregnant, then those particular oils would be avoided.

And finally, the order of blending is important too. This has a lot to do with the chemical characteristics of the oils you are going to use. An essential oil that possesses very strong properties may need to be diluted by the characteristic of other essential oils to achieve the effect you want, so it should be added first. It is a good idea to study the different characteristics of the oils you propose using before you commence making your blend.

I have included a useful table on the following two pages to help you with your blends.

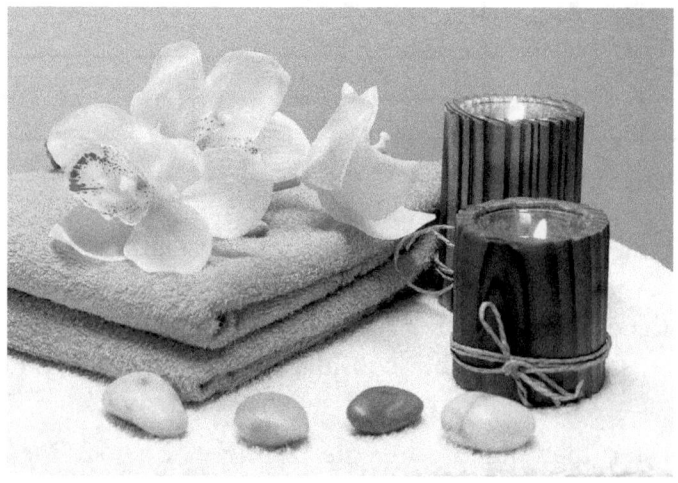

Oil	Note	Intensity	Blends With
Citrus			
Bergamot	Top	Low	Chamomile, Clary Sage, Geranium, Jasmine, Lavender, Neroli, Rose
Grapefruit	Top	Low	Clove, Geranium, Jasmine, Lavender, Lemon, Neroli, Rosemary
Lemon	Top	Low	Eucalyptus, Frankincense, Geranium, Lavender, Myrrh, Rose, Sandalwood, Ylang Ylang
Mandarin	Top	Low	Cinnamon, Clove, Grapefruit, Lavender, Tangerine
Floral			
Chamomile	Middle	High	Bergamot, Cedarwood, Clary Sage, Geranium, Lavender, Rose, Sandalwood,
Helichrysum	Middle	High	Grapefruit, Lavender, Lemon, Mandarin, Rose
Jasmine	Middle	High	Bergamot, Clary Sage, Grapefruit, Rose, Sandalwood, Ylang Ylang
Neroli	Middle	High	Bergamot, Grapefruit, Jasmine, Lemon, Mandarin, Rose
Rose	Middle	High	Bergamot, Clary Sage, Clove, Geranium, Jasmine, Lavender, Ylang Ylang
Ylang Ylang	Middle	High	Geranium, Grapefruit, Jasmine, Neroli, Orange, Sandalwood
Herbaceous			
Clary Sage	Middle	Medium	Bergamot, Frankincense, Geranium, Grapefruit, Lavender, Lemon, Pine, Sweet Orange
Geranium	Middle	Medium	Bergamot, Clove, Lavender, Lemon, Grapefruit, Patchouli, Sandalwood, Sweet Orange
Lavender	Middle	Medium	Bergamot, Clary Sage, Frankincense, Geranium, Grapefruit, Lemon, Patchouli, Pine, Rose, Rosemary, Sweet Orange
Marjoram	Middle	Medium	Bergamot, Chamomile, Lavender, Lemon, Peppermint, Tea Tree, Thyme
Pine	Middle	Medium	Bergamot, Frankincense, Lavender, Lemon, Rosemary, Tea Tree
Thyme	Middle	Medium	Bergamot, Clary Sage, Grapefruit, Lavender, Lemon, Marjoram, Tea Tree

Oil	Note	Intensity	Blends With
Camphorous			
Eucalyptus	Top	High	Lavender, Lemon, Lemongrass, Peppermint, Rosemary, Thyme
Peppermint	Top	High	Eucalyptus, Lavender, Lemon, Mandarin, Marjoram, Rosemary
Rosemary	Middle	Medium	Bergamot, Cinnamon, Frankincense, Lemon, Peppermint, Pine
Tea Tree	Top	High	Clary Sage, Eucalyptus, Geranium, Lavender, Lemon, Pine, Ylang Ylang
Spice			
Cinnamon	Middle	High	Geranium, Grapefruit, Lavender, Lemon, Mandarin, Sandalwood
Clove	Middle	Medium	Bergamot, Chamomile, Clary Sage, Geranium, Grapefruit, Jasmine, Lavender, Rose, Ylang Ylang
Wood and Resin			
Frankincense	Base	High	Geranium, Grapefruit, Lavender, Lemon, Mandarin, Rose, Sandalwood
Myrrh	Base	High	Frankincense, Geranium, Lavender, Lemongrass, Mandarin, Patchouli, Pine, Rose
Patchouli	Base	High	Clary Sage, Geranium, Lavender, Myrrh, Rose, Sandalwood
Sandalwood	Base	Low	Bergamot, Clove, Frankincense, Geranium, Lavender, Myrrh, Patchouli, Rose, Ylang Ylang

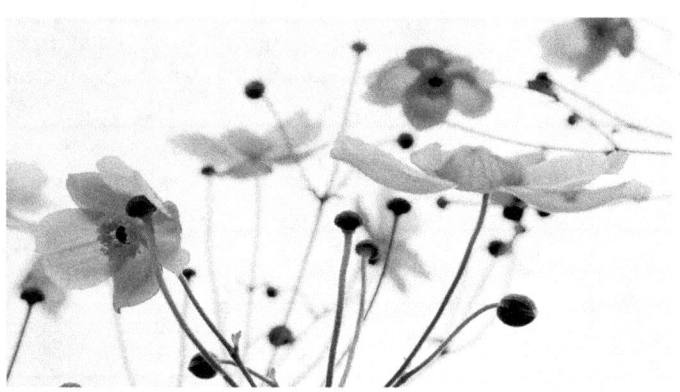

9. Diluting Essential Oils

It can be a bad idea to apply essential oils directly to the skin. In some cases it can cause burns or irritation in cases of sensitive skin.

Having said that, in certain instances tea tree and lavender can be used "neat", however, in some individuals, they can cause burns, so it is always best to play safe and dilute all essential oils in a carrier oil.

Also, "watch the drops" As mentioned earlier in this book, if a recipe specifies two drops, then that is what you should use. Doubling the quantity up to four drops, does not make for a better blend. In fact doubling up in this way could cause a very significant unwanted reaction. So watch the dilutions!

Below is a useful table for percentage dilutions and uses, and on the following page I have included a table to help you calculate dilutions.

Dilution And Uses	
Dilution	**Uses**
1%	For sensitive skin, children, the elderly, health condition, massages
2%	Standard dilution for most purposes especially whole body massage
4%	For massaging specific areas of the body
5%	For short term use for muscle pains and respiratory system conditions such as congestion.
10%	Provides temporary relief for specific health conditions
25%	Provides short term relief for cramps, severe pain

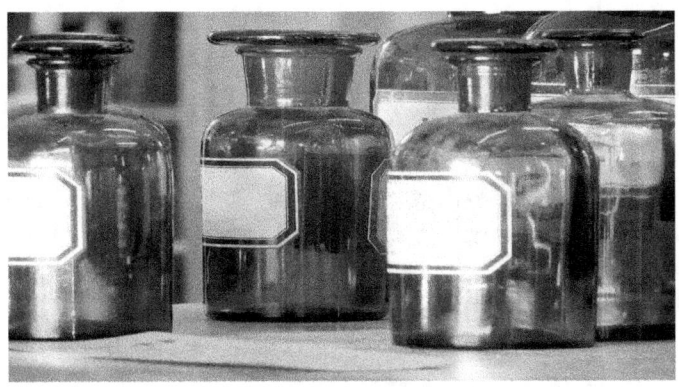

Carrier Oil	Essential Oil % Dilution And (Drops)					
By Volume	1%	2%	4%	5%	10%	25%
1/8th oz.						
1/2 Teaspoon	(1)	(2)	(4)	(5)	(10)	(25)
5ml						
1/4 oz..						
1 Teaspoon	(2)	(4)	(8)	(10)	(20)	(50)
10ml						
1/2 oz.						
1 Tablespoon	(3)	(6)	(12)	(15)	(30)	(75)
15ml						
1 oz.						
2 Tablespoons	(6)	(12)	(24)	(30)	(60)	(150)
30ml						
2 oz.						
4 Tablespoons	(12)	(24)	(48)	(60)	(120)	(300)
60ml						

As you can see from the above table, ounces and milliliters do not convert equally into each other. Therefore, use either ounces or milliliters, do not try and use both in the same dilution.

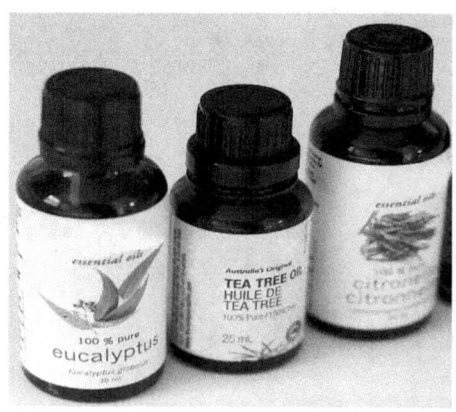

10. Carrier Oils

Carrier oils are a necessity in aromatherapy, and there are many different types available, such as sweet almond oil, apricot kernel oil, jojoba oil, borage seed oil—borage oil is rich in omega 6 essential fatty acids which the body does not manufacture itself, but must be obtained from the diet.

Other carrier oils include evening primrose oil—also an omega 6 essential fatty acid—grapeseed oil, Olive Oil and sunflower oil to name a few. Look for organic cold pressed varieties. Being cold pressed—in other words, no heat has been used—means that all the goodness is retained in the oil. This could mean not just the natural fragrance, but any vitamins and minerals as well.

It is not advisable to use the oils you keep in the kitchen cupboard for cooking purposes. These oils are usually heat treated and refined in a different way to what we need for aromatherapy purposes.

How To Use Essential Oils

Okay, you have now mixed some essential oils—either blends or single oils—so how do you use them? There are several methods that you can employ, depending on the purpose you are using the essential oils for.

Diffusion

There are different ways that essential oils can be diffused.

Candle Diffusion. In this method a candle is lit in the base of the unit which warms the oil which has been placed in a tray on top of the unit. The aromas from the oil are them dispersed into the room.

Clay Pots. With this method no heat is used. The oil is stored in the pot. The aroma from the oil is released into the room by removing the stopper from the pot. These pots are often made from terra-cotta.

Fan Diffusers. Again, heat is not used with a fan diffuser. The essential oil is deposited on to an absorbent pad which is them placed inside the fan. Cold air blowing over the pad picks up the aroma which is them dispersed into the room. These units can be either electric or battery powered. Make sure you get one large enough for the room that it is to be sited in.

Lamp Ring. Lamp rings are made from terra-cotta. They are placed on the light bulb. A ring on the lamp contains a groove into which the essential oil is placed. The heat from the bulb warms the ring which them heats the oil. The aroma from the oil is them dispersed into the room.

Nebulizer. This heat diffusion method is the most expensive and a very effective way of dispersing essential oils into a room. The unit consists of an electric base unit which incorporates a pump and an atomizer. Some nebulizers use glass tubing instead, however, the principle is still the same. The beauty of this unit is that no heat is involved. The pump pushes the essential oil through the atomizer or glass tubes which is then converted into microscopic particles which are then expelled into the room. Many different models are available, and at different price points, so make sure that you purchase one that will be suitable for the size of the room you propose putting it in.

Ingestion.

As mentioned elsewhere in this book, it is a bad idea to ingest essential oils except under the supervision of a trained and qualified aromatherapist or doctor.

Topical Applications.

One of the most effective ways to apply essential oils is to use some of the ways listed below, to allow the essential oils to ingest through the skin. They provide many benefits for health and well-being. Essential oils are easily applied as first aid remedies. Helichrysum and chamomile possess anti-inflammatory properties which make them useful for reducing localized inflammation. Eucalyptus and tea tree possess anti-bacterial and antiviral properties which make them useful for strengthening the immune system and counteracting the effects of colds, flu and sinusitis.

Bath.

Adding essential oils to bath water can provide tremendous relief for stress, relaxation or for various health concerns. Into a carrier oil add six to eight drops (in total) of your chosen oils. The carrier oil will help to disperse the essential oils in the water. Citrus and spice essential oils as well as peppermint can be irritating in bath water to some individuals. Adding essential oils to bath water can help the respiratory system as well as being beneficial for stress and insomnia. Warm water increases the absorption of the oils through the skin.

Sitz Bath.

This means using a few inches of water in the bath—just enough to cover the lower body. Sitz baths can be very effective for hemorrhoids, yeast infections in men and women and painful periods. They are also good for irritations or infections of the urinary, genital and rectum areas of the body.

Massage.

You can achieve good therapeutic benefits by massaging essential oils directly into the skin. This technique can be done to relieve stress or anxiety, for relaxation or for various health reasons. A massage can be applied to the whole body or localized areas. Try 2 to 3% essential oils of your choices diluted with vegetable, nut or a seed carrier oil, or unscented natural lotion or cream. A 4% dilution (24 drops) can be used for localized areas of the body needing a more intensive concentration.

Compress.

A cold compress will reduce inflammation by dispersing heat from the affected area. A hot compress increases blood flow to the affected area. A hot compress will ease pain, reduce congestion, draw out pus and be a relaxant in cases of spasms. Mix your essential oil selection with water. Soak the cloth and wring out. Apply the compress to the affected area. Repeat as needed.

Creams and Lotions.

Buy unscented creams and add essential oils as required.

Inhaling.

Inhaling diluted essential oils is beneficial for various respiratory system conditions including congestion, colds, cough, flu and infection of the sinuses. Prepare a bowl of boiling water and add 5-10 drops of your chosen essential oil to the water. Cover your head with a towel and breathe in the vapors through the nose. It is best to keep your eyes closed to avoid any eye irritation. Additionally, apply drops of diluted essential oil to a handkerchief or cotton ball and breathe in the aroma.

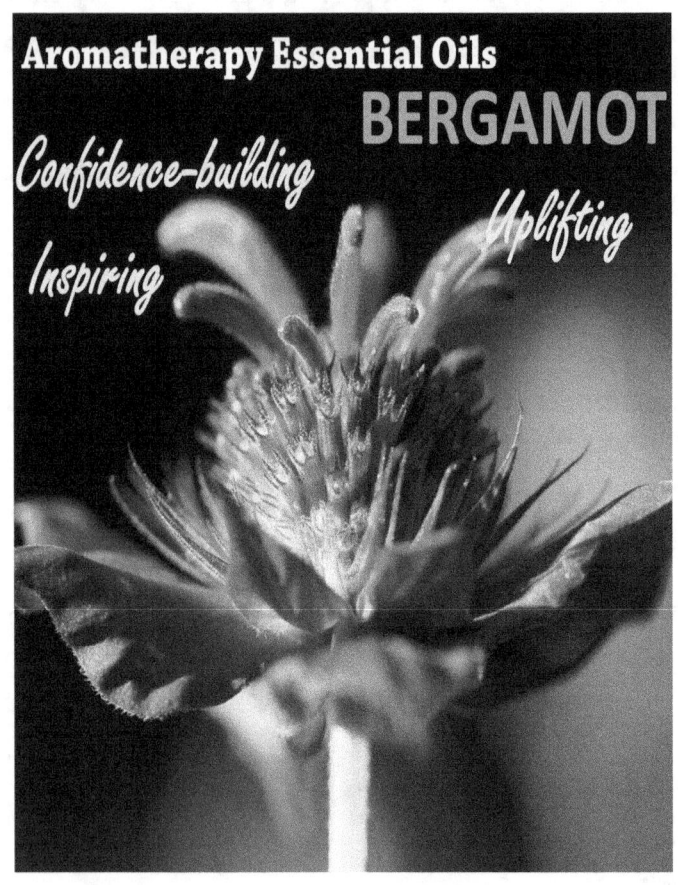

11. Essential Oil Profiles

Latin Names and Chemistry

It is very important to become familiar with the Latin name of the plants from which the essential oil is derived. Why is this and is it not too difficult to understand all these strange names? Not at all! Knowing what the Latin names of various plants are from which essential oils are extracted will ensure that you are getting the correct essential oil for the treatment that you envision doing. Also remember, that many plants have very similar common names, and it is so easy to get the wrong oil.

Bergamot

Latin Name: *Citrus bergamia*

Note: Top

Odor Intensity: Low

Parts Used: Peel

Extracted By: Cold Pressed

Comes from: Algeria, Italy, Ivory Coast, Morocco, Tunisia

Dilution: Dilute as desired. Can be used topically or use in a diffuser.

Description:

Bergamot is named after the city of Bergamo in Italy where the oil was originally sold. In addition, Bergamot is used to flavor Earl Grey tea.

Bergamot has many uses. For example, in skin care products it can be added to lotions to treat acne and eczema. It can also be used to detoxify the skin and added to a compress to draw out a boil. It is also used for digestive problems—add a drop to black tea to counteract bloating and flatulence. Bergamot also provides urinary system support—especially for cystitis, and when added to a sitz bath it helps prevent the spread of infection from the urethra to the bladder. Bergamot possesses an uplifting ability and is therefore useful for anxiety, stress and other emotional problems.

Precautions: Bergamot can cause phototoxicity and irritation to the skin. Therefore, avoid direct sunlight for a period of at least 12 hours after use.

Blends well with the majority of other oils, notably:

Cypress	Clary Sage	Frankincense
Geranium	Lavender	Sage

Used for::

Anxiety	Bladder Problems
Depression	Digestive Problems, Bloating, Flatulence
Eczema	Sleep Disorders
Herpes Simplex Virus Type 1 (Cold Sores)	

Chamomile—Roman

Latin name: *Chamaemlum nobile*

Note: Middle

Odor Intensity: Very high

Parts Used: Flowers and leaves

Extracted By: Steam Distillation

Comes From: Bulgaria, Chile, France, Hungary, Italy, United Kingdom, United States, Yugoslavia

Dilution: Dilute as desired. Can be used topically, diffused or directly inhaled.

Description:

Used for thousands of years in Europe, it is a great aid for the nervous system—especially for stress, fear and anxiety. It can be burned in an Aromalamp at night to relieve restlessness and insomnia. It also has excellent anti-inflammatory properties in addition to it being a good urinary tract disinfectant.

Taken internally as a tea or tincture, it provides support for the digestive system for such conditions as bloating, flatulence and other disorders caused by anxiety and tension. In addition, it is also a useful aid for liver congestion.

Chamomile can be added to skin lotions to treat acne, eczema, psoriasis, rashes, dermatitis in addition to helping with wound healing and soothing the effects of sunburn.

Precautions: If you are allergic to ragweed, then, you may be allergic to chamomile.

Blends with:

Bergamot	Clary sage	Jasmine	Lavender
Lemon	Neroli	Rose	Sandalwood

Used For:
Digestive System Disorders,
Nervous System Disorders
Skin Disorders: Acne, Eczema, Psoriasis, Rashes, Wound Healing, Sunburn

Cinnamon

Latin Name: *Cinnamomum zeylanicum*

Note: Middle

Odor Intensity: High

Parts Used: Bark, leaves

Extracted By: Steam Distillation

Comes From: Africa, Burma, Comoro Islands, India, Indo-China, Jamaica, Madagascar, Sri Lanka

Dilution: Diluted as desired with carrier oil. Can be diffused or inhaled.

Description:

There are two varieties of cinnamon—cinnamon leaf and cinnamon bark. In each case the oil is extracted by a steam/water distillation process. Cinnamon bark is a lot stronger than the leaf variety, and as such, it can be an irritant when used for massage purposes. Cinnamon leaf is more therapeutic and is used for disorders of the digestive system, circulatory system and as a support for the immune system. As it provides a warming effect, it is an excellent treatment for colds and flu symptoms when rubbed onto the chest area.

Both oils are a good choice as antibacterials, antifungals and antivirals, and can be used to destroy intestinal parasites.

Precautions: Always use diluted cinnamon essential oil. Both derivatives can be irritating to the skin. Anyone who is taking a blood thinning medication as well as pregnant women and small children should not use cinnamon essential oils.

Blends with:
Frankincense Mandarin   Sweet Orange   Ylang Ylang

Used For:
Colds and Flu, Intestinal Parasites, Bacterial, Fungal and Viral Infections,
Circulatory System Problems,
Digestive System Problems
Immune System Support

Clary Sage

Latin Name: *Salvia sclarea*

Note: Middle

Odor Intensity: Medium

Parts Used: Flowering Tops / Leaves

Extracted By: Steam Distillation

Comes From: Bulgaria, England, France, Germany, Italy, Morocco, Russia, Spain, United States

Dilution: Dilute as desired. Can be used topically or use in a diffuser.

Description:

Used for thousands of years in Europe to treat nervous system problems, and also for its euphoric and intoxicating results, therefore, clary sage should only be used in moderation. In more modern times, clary sage is used as a treatment for menstrual problems including cramping, hot flashes, overdue or sporadic flow and PMS. Clary Sage possesses antispasmodic properties which makes it useful in the treatment of asthma as well as strained muscles.

Precautions: Avoid consuming alcohol while using clary sage as it may increase the potency of the alcohol. Avoid using whilst pregnant. Do not use if you have low blood pressure or estrogen dependent tumors.

Blends With:

Bergamot	Frankincense	Geranium	Lavender
Pine	Patchouli	Rose	Sandalwood

Used For:
Nervous system disorders
Menstrual problems
Respiratory problems
Muscle strain

Clove Bud

Latin Name: *Eugenia caryophyllata*

Note: Middle

Odor Intensity: Medium

Parts Used: Unopened Flowers

Extracted By: Steam Distillation

Comes From: Indonesia, Madagascar, Molucca Islands, Philippines, Sri Lanka, Tanzania, West Indies

Dilution: Dilute as desired. Can be used topically or use in a diffuser.

Description:

A powerful antiseptic and anesthetic, clove can be used in small amounts in a diffuser or inhaler to fight the common cold. It is also good in the digestive system to stimulate the digestion process. In addition, it is also effective to eliminate intestinal parasites. Always dilute clove—do not use it neat.

Precautions: Do not use if you are taking blood thinners as clove can reduce blood clotting. Clove can cause skin irritation which can result in dermatitis. Only use in a diffuser for a few minutes at a time otherwise eye irritation may occur.

Blends With:

Bergamot	Cinnamon	Clary Sage	Geranium
Lavender	Lemon	Mandarin	Rosemary
Sandalwood			

Used For:
Colds
Digestive System Problems
Intestinal Parasites
Oral Infections
Toothache

Eucalyptus

Latin Name: *Eucalyptus globulus*

Note: Top

Odor Intensity: Very High

Parts Used: Leaves

Extracted By: Steam Distillation

Comes From: Australia, Bolivia, Brazil, China, Ecuador, Portugal, Russia, Spain, United States (California)

Dilution: Dilute as desired. Can be used topically, diffused or directly inhaled.

Description:

Eucalyptus supports the respiratory system as it is a very powerful decongestant and expectorant. It is best used as an inhaler for colds, catarrh and general respiratory system problems. Use Eucalyptus in a diffuser to help prevent the spread of respiratory infections.

Mixed with massage oil, eucalyptus can be used as a chest rub to ease a chest infection. In addition, it can also be used in this way to ease muscle strains. When applied to a wound dressing, it will hasten the healing process.

Precautions: Do not use if you have epilepsy or high blood pressure. Use in moderation on the skin. Eucalyptus may compromise homeopathic remedies.

Blends With:

Chamomile	Geranium	Grapefruit	Juniper
Lavender	Lemon	Peppermint	

Used For:
Respiratory System infections such as: Bronchitis, Colds, Coughs
Herpes Simplex Virus (Chicken Pox)
Insect Repellent
Intestinal Parasites
Muscle Strains
Sinus Congestion

Frankincense

Latin Name: *Boswellia carteri*

Note: Base

Odor Intensity: High

Parts Used: Resin

Extracted By: Steam Distillation

Comes From: China, Ethiopia, Oman, Saudi Arabia, Somalia

Dilution: Dilute as desired with carrier oil. Can be used topically, diffused or directly inhaled.

Description:

Used since ancient times, but perhaps best known as a gift to the new born Jesus along with gold and myrrh. It is used for the respiratory system—by means of steam inhalation— for such conditions as bronchitis and severe colds. It can also be used as a gargle for a sore throat or to release catarrh. In the urinary system it is used for urinary tract infections. It is also used beneficially as a douche for symptoms of PMS and other menstrual problems.

And finally, it is a useful addition to creams or lotions to aid in chapped skin conditions. In addition, it is also useful for boils, pimples and other skin conditions.

Precautions: Do not use if you are pregnant.

Blends With:

Bergamot	Clary Sage	Cinnamon	Coriander
Geranium	Grapefruit	Lavender	Lemon
Mandarin	Neroli	Patchouli	Pine
Rose	Sandalwood	Ylang Ylang	

Used For:
Respiratory System Problems
Urinary System Problems
Skin Problems
Wound Healing

Geranium

Latin Name: *Pelargonium graveolens*

Note: Middle

Odor Intensity: High

Parts Used: Leaves / Flower Heads

Extracted By: Steam Distillation

Comes From: Algeria, China, Egypt, France, Madagascar, Morocco, Russia, South Africa, United States

Dilution: Dilute as desired. Can be used topically, diffused or directly inhaled.

Description:

The pelargonium variety is most often used in aromatherapy. Its uplifting fragrance supplies support to the nervous system for such conditions as anxiety and depression. It is also an excellent skin tonic especially for such conditions as acne, eczema and wound healing, also for relieving blisters associated with the Herpes Simplex virus type 1. Geranium essential oil is also useful for regulating hormones and is therefore a good treatment for PMS, menopausal symptoms and other menstruation issues.

Precautions: Do not use neat on the skin as it can cause skin irritation. Do not use if pregnant. Do not consume internally as it can have a negative effect with some medications.

Blends with:

Bergamot	Chamomile	Clary Sage	Clove
Frankincense	Ginger	Grapefruit	Jasmine
Lavender	Lemon	Mandarin	Neroli
Patchouli	Peppermint	Rose	Rosemary

Used For:
Nervous system problems
Skin conditions
Balances hormones

Ginger

Latin Name: *Zingiber officinale*

Note: Middle

Odor Density: Medium

Parts Used: Rhizome

Extracted By: Steam Distillation

Comes From: India, Indonesia, China, Nepal, Nigeria, Thailand

Dilution: Dilute as desired. Can be used topically, diffused or directly inhaled.

Description:

Ginger has been used for centuries for a variety of health conditions, but it is best known as a treatment for morning sickness, and motion sickness, as well as feelings of nausea generally. It is also used as a treatment for colds, congestion, coughs sore throat, cramp, fever, muscle strains and arthritis. Studies show that ginger essential oil is toxic to prostate and lung cancer cells, but not breast cancer cells.

Precautions: May cause skin irritation.

Blends With:

Bergamot   Clove Eucalyptus   Frankincense Geranium
Grapefruit   Jasmine   Lemon   Mandarin   Neroli
Patchouli   Rose   Sandalwood   Ylang Ylang

Used For:
Digestive System Support
Respiratory System Support
Arthritis
Muscle strains
Certain cancers

Grapefruit, Pink

Latin Name: *Citrus paradise*

Note: Top

Odor Intensity: Medium

Parts Used: Peel

Extracted By: Cold Pressed

Comes From: Brazil, Israel, South Africa, United States (California, Florida)

Dilution: Dilute as desired. Can be used topically, diffused or directly inhaled.

Description:

Grapefruit essential oil provides balance and tone to the digestive system. It also supplies support for the nervous system in cases of depression and anxiety. This essential oil creates a "happy feeling" and is therefore useful where stressful situations are involved.

Grapefruit essential oil is also useful in cases of inadequate removal of toxins from the body, such as cellulite (dilute in massage oil), lymphatic drainage and fluid retention. It is also useful for various skin conditions including acne, and oily skin. It also provides support for the circulatory system as well as being a liver tonic.

Precautions: Grapefruit essential oil has a very short shelf life; therefore only small quantities should be purchased at a time. Always dilute in a carrier oil or lotion. Of all the citrus oils, this one is the least sensitive to sunlight. Can be an irritant to sensitive skin.

Blends With:

Bergamot	Clary Sage	Clove Eucalyptus	Frankincense
Geranium	Ginger	Lavender	Lemon
Mandarin	Neroli	Patchouli	Peppermint
Rosemary	Thyme	Ylang Ylang	

Used For:

Circulatory System Support   Digestive System Support
Nervous System Support   Removal of Toxins from the Body
Skin Conditions

Helichrysum

Latin Name: *Helichrysum italicum*

Note: Middle

Odor Intensity: High

Parts Used: Flowers

Extracted By: Steam Distillation

Comes From: Corsica, France, Hungary, Italy, Spain

Dilution: Dilute as desired. Can be used topically, diffused or directly inhaled.

Description:

Assists the body to fight any infection caused by a weak immune system—such as allergies and infections. Excellent for treating the effects of a cold or flu. This essential oil is also used for treating skin conditions such as bruises, burns, dry and cracked skin, eczema, psoriasis and wound healing. In the respiratory system it is used as a decongestant to treat asthma and bronchitis. Can be used in massage oil for rheumatism and muscle strains.

Precautions: Do not take internally. Do not use if pregnant.

Blends With:

Chamomile	Eucalyptus	Frankincense	Geranium
Grapefruit	Lavender	Lemon	Mandarin
Neroli	Pine	Rose	Rosemary
Tea tree	Thyme	Ylang Ylang	

Used For:

Respiratory System Support
Immune System Support
Skin Problems
Rheumatism
Muscle Strains

Jasmine

Latin Name: *Jasminum officinale, Jasminum grandiflorum*

Note: Base

Odor Intensity: High

Parts Used: Flower

Extracted By: Solvent Extraction

Comes From: Algeria, China, Egypt, France, India, Morocco

Dilution: Dilute as desired. Can be used topically, diffused or directly inhaled.

Description:

Jasmine is often associated with a heady fragrance in the evening and at night. It is one of the most expensive oils as several different processes are involved in its extraction. Only the flowers are used and these have to be picked at night when the fragrance is most concentrated—this also adds to the cost. It takes over 3 million flowers to produce one pound of oil. And because it is so expensive, there are many adulterated products on the market. If you are offered cheap Jasmine essential oil, then, chances are it is not the real thing, so beware!

Jasmine provides support to the nervous system in cases of depression and nervous tension. In addition it is used during labor to strengthen uterine contractions. It is also used to ease cramps and spasms during uncomfortable periods, as well as supplying prostate support for men.

Jasmine also supports the respiratory system in cases of coughs and laryngitis. When burnt in an Aromalamp it provides an excellent treatment for sexual dysfunction including impotence and premature ejaculation. Jasmine essential oil is known as an aphrodisiac. It is also a good skin toner for such conditions as eczema and dry and irritated skin as it is a balancer of sebum which makes it suitable for all skin types.

Precautions: Do not ingest. Because of its high cost, watch out for adulterated products. Do not use if pregnant or breastfeeding. Can cause skin sensitivity in some individuals.

Jasmine (Cont'd)

Blends With:

Bergamot	Clary Sage	Clove	Coriander
Geranium	Ginger	Grapefruit	Lemon
Mandarin	Neroli	Patchouli	Rose
Sandalwood	Ylang Ylang		

Used For:

Nervous System Support
Respiratory System Support
Sexual Dysfunction
Uterine Contractions
Period Pains

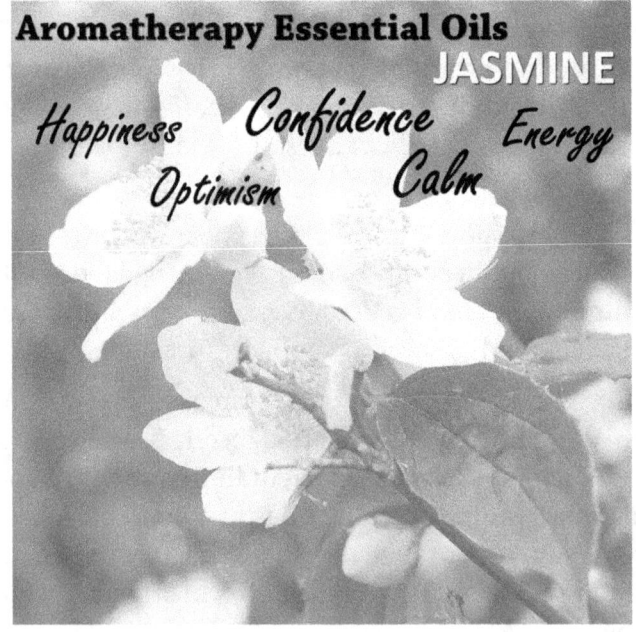

Lavender

Latin Name: *Lavandula* angustifolia

Note: Middle

Odor Intensity: Medium

Parts Used: Flowering Tops and Leaves

Extracted By: Steam Distillation

Comes From: Bulgaria, China, Croatia, England, France, Russia, Tasmania, Yugoslavia

Dilution: Dilute as desired. Can be used topically, diffused or directly inhaled.

Description:

If you can only afford to buy one essential oil then choose lavender, as it is one of the most versatile essential oils available. It supplies support to the respiratory system for such conditions as asthma, bronchitis, colds and throat infections. For the nervous system it provides support in cases of anxiety, depression, stress, headaches, insomnia and migraines.

Lavender is also a good skin treatment for acne, boils sunburn, psoriasis and—for one of its most common uses— healing of burns and wounds. In the digestive system it is a good treatment for colic, bloating, flatulence and nausea. It is also useful in cases of rheumatism, arthritis and muscle strains. It also stimulates the immune system to work effectively.

Precautions: Be caution if you use lavender whilst pregnant. Make sure that you purchase true lavender (*Lavandula angustifolia*). There are many lavender derivatives on the market which can give unwanted or unknown contraindications.

Blends With:

Bergamot	Clary Sage	Clove	Eucalyptus	Pine
Frankincense	Geranium	Chamomile	Grapefruit	Lemon
Lemongrass	Mandarin	Jasmine	Patchouli	Thyme

Used For:

Digestive System Support   Nervous System Support
Respiratory System Support   Immune System Support
Skin Problems   Arthritis   Rheumatism   Muscle Strains

Lemon

Latin Name: *Citrus limonum*

Note: Top

Odor Intensity: Low

Parts Used: Peel

Extracted By: Cold Pressed

Comes From: Argentina, Brazil, Cyprus, Guinea, Israel, Italy, Portugal, Sicily, Spain, United States (California and Florida)

Dilution: Dilute as desired. Can be used topically, diffused or directly inhaled.

Description:

It takes roughly 1,500 lemons to make one pound of essential oil. Mixed with water, lemon makes a really good liver cleansing drink. Lemon essential oil mixed with massage oil and then rubbed into the belly helps in the liver detoxification process. Lemon essential oil provides support to the immune system by helping build white blood cells which are part of the body's defenses against unwanted pathogens which can cause serious problems in the body. Lemon essential oil also assists in the formation of red blood cells and can help support the circulatory system—especially in cases of arteriosclerosis. Lemon mixed in water provides an important heart tonic.

Lemon essential oil provides support to the digestive system. When taken internally it has an alkalizing effect which can help maintain the pH of the body. The majority of people in the United States and Europe has a very acidic body—often called acidosis. This is a result of consuming the typical Western diet which is high in saturated fat. An acidic body can lead to inflammation—arthritis and rheumatism in the joints. Drinking lemon in water can alleviate some of the pain of these conditions.

Lemon essential oil also provides support to the respiratory system and as such is a useful treatment for asthma, bronchitis, colds, cough sore throat and flu.

Precautions: Lemon essential oil has a short shelf life. May irritate sensitive skin. Avoid sunlight after using the oil on the skin. Only use low concentrations of the oil.

Lemon (Cont'd)

Blends With:

Bergamot	Cinnamon	Clary Sage	Clove Eucalyptus
Frankincense	Geranium	Chamomile	Grapefruit
Lavender	Lemongrass	Mandarin	Neroli
Patchouli	Rose	Sandalwood	Ylang Ylang

Used For:

Circulatory System Support
Digestive System Support
Immune System Support
Respiratory System Support
pH Body Balancing

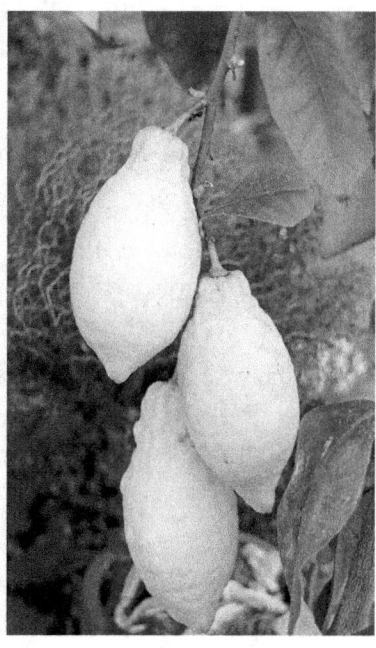

Aromatherapy
Essential Oils

LEMON

Clarity   Positivity
Energy
Motivation   Calm
Concentration

Lemongrass

Latin Name: *Cymbopogon flexuosus*

Note: Top

Oder Intensity: Medium

Parts Used: Leaves

Extracted By: Steam Distillation

Comes From: Brazil, Guatemala, India, Madagascar, Nepal, Sri Lanka

Dilution: Dilute as desired with carrier oil. Use in a diffuser, directly inhale or apply topically

Description:

Supports the nervous system by reducing stress and depression. It also supports the circulatory system and helps purge lactic acid and therefore is useful for athletes as it will ease muscle aches and pains.

Lemongrass is also a useful antibacterial and antifungal and as such is a useful treatment for athlete's foot, or any other fungal or bacterial infection. Lemongrass also supports the respiratory system in cases of colds, cough, laryngitis and sore throat. Lemongrass is also an excellent skin tonic as well as being an insect repellent.

Precautions: Lemongrass may cause skin irritation in people with sensitive skin. Only use one or two drops when diluting the oil. Lemongrass oil should not be used if pregnant

Blends With:

Bergamot	Clary Sage	Coriander	Geranium
Ginger	Grapefruit	Lavender	Lemon
Marjoram	Patchouli	Rosemary	Tea Tree
Thyme	Ylang Ylang		

Used For:
Supports the Circulatory System
Supports the Nervous System
Supports the Respiratory System
Skin Tonic
Antibacterial
Antifungal

Mandarin Green or Red

Latin Name: *Citrus reticulata*

Note: Top

Odor Intensity: Low (Green)—Medium to High (Red)

Parts Used: Peel

Extracted By: Cold pressed

Comes From: Brazil, Italy, Algeria, Tunisia, Spain, Cyprus, Greece, Argentina, China

Dilution: Dilute as desired. Can be used topically, diffused or directly inhaled.

Description:

This very gentle oil makes an excellent skin tonic for the young and elderly. It helps with wrinkles, stretch marks, scars, acne, oily skin and age spots. Mandarin essential oil also provides excellent support for the digestive system. It assists in expelling gas from the intestines helps relieve cramps and spasms and can be used for babies who have colic. In addition, it aids bile production and helps relieve constipation.

Blends With:

Chamomile	Cinnamon	Clary Sage	Clove
Frankincense	Geranium	Grapefruit	Jasmine
Lemon	Myrrh	Neroli	Patchouli
Rose	Sandalwood	Ylang Ylang	

Used For:

Digestive System Support
Skin Problems

Marjoram, Sweet

Latin Name: *Origanum majorana*

Note: Middle

Odor Intensity: Medium

Parts Used: Leaves / Flowering Tops

Extracted By: Steam Distillation

Comes From: Bulgaria, Egypt, France, Germany, Hungary, Morocco, Portugal, Spain, Tunisia, Yugoslavia

Dilution: Dilute as desired with carrier oil. Diffuse, directly inhale or apply topically

Description:

Marjoram provides support for the respiratory system in cases of asthma, cough, colds, flu and respiratory conditions in general. It also supply support for the immune system. Marjoram also supports the digestive system for such problems as intestinal cramps, diarrhea, flatulence, indigestion and constipation.

Diluted in massage oil, marjoram is ideal for treating arthritis, bruises, joint pain and rheumatism. Marjoram also supports the nervous system by calming nerves and releasing tension. It is also an excellent choice for anyone suffering from insomnia.

Precautions: Do not use if pregnant. May reduce sexual craving

Blends With:

Bergamot	Chamomile	Clary Sage	Eucalyptus
Geranium	Lavender	Lemon	Neroli
Peppermint	Pine	Rosemary	Tea Tree
Thyme Linalol			

Used For:
Digestive System Support
Nervous System Support
Respiratory System Support
Arthritis
Joint Pain
Rheumatism
Insomnia

Myrrh

Latin Name: *Commiphora myrrha*

Note: Base

Odor Intensity: High

Parts Used: Resin

Extracted By: Steam Distillation

Comes From: Africa, Arabia, Ethiopia, Somalia, Sudan, Yemen

Dilution: Dilute as desired. Can be used topically, diffused or directly inhaled.

Description:

Myrrh supplies powerful support for the respiratory system. It has drying and cleansing abilities which assist in eliminating infection as well as expelling mucus following an attack of bronchitis, a cold or cough. It also helps in cases of asthma.

Myrrh can also be added to massage oil which is then applied to the abdomen to assist the digestive system in cases of indigestion, flatulence and diarrhea.

Eczema, boils and infected wounds can all be relieved with myrrh essential oil. And because it possesses antifungal properties, it is also a good treatment for athlete's foot.

Added to skincare cream myrrh provides support for dry and chapped skin, as well as skin that is aging prematurely.

Precautions: Do not use if pregnant. Exercise caution if you have low blood sugar.

Blends With:

Bergamot	Cinnamon	Clove	Eucalyptus	Frankincense
Geranium	Grapefruit	Lemon	Mandarin	Patchouli
Peppermint	Pine	Chamomile		Rosemary
Sandalwood	Lavender			

Used For:

Digestive System Support
Respiratory System Support
Skin Problems
Antifungal—Athlete's Foot

Neroli

Latin Name: *Citrus aurantium*

Note: Middle

Odor Intensity: Medium

Parts Used: Flowers

Extracted By: Steam Distillation

Comes From: Algeria, Egypt, France, Italy, Morocco, Tunisia, United States (California)

Dilution: Dilute as desired. Can be used topically, diffused or directly inhaled.

Description:

Derived from the flowers of the Seville orange tree using steam distillation, neroli has an exquisite scent which when a few drops are added to bath water provides a very relaxing experience. Neroli supports the nervous system for such conditions as anxiety, stress and feelings of hopelessness. For the skin it has cell rejuvenating properties for skin that is aging prematurely.

Neroli also provides support for the digestive system for conditions such as indigestion and diarrhea caused by nervous conditions. It also assists in expelling gas from the intestines. Neroli is also considered one of the best oils to enhance sexual desire due to its gentle fragrance.

Precautions: Considered safe

Blends With:

Clary Sage	Coriander	Frankincense	Geranium
Ginger	Grapefruit	Jasmine	Lavender
Lemon	Mandarin	Chamomile	Rose
Sandalwood	Ylang Ylang		

Used For:
Nervous System Support
Skin Conditions
Sexual Desire

Orange, Bitter

Latin Name: *Citrus aurantium*

Note: Top

Odor Intensity: Medium

Parts Used: Peel

Extracted By: Cold Pressed

Comes From: Italy, Spain, United States

Dilution: Dilute as desired with carrier oil. Diffuse or apply topically.

Description:

When ephedra was banned for use in weight loss products in the United States and Europe, supplement manufacturers started using bitter orange as a substitute appetite suppressant ingredient in their products. In addition, bitter orange supports the digestive system in cases of indigestion, and as a liver stimulant.

Precautions: May cause irritation to someone who has a sensitive skin. Do not go out in sunlight for at least 12 hours after using this product, as it has phototoxic properties.

Blends With:

Bergamot	Clary Sage	Frankincense	Ginger
Grapefruit	Lavender	Lemon	Mandarin
Myrrh	Neroli		

Used For:

Digestive System Support

Appetite Suppressant—Weight Loss

Orange, Sweet

Latin Name: *Citrus sinensis*

Note: Top

Odor Intensity: Medium

Parts Used: Peel

Extracted By: Cold Pressed

Comes From: Italy, South Africa, Spain, United States

Dilution: Dilute as desired with carrier oil. May be diffused, inhaled directly or applied topically

Description:

Orange oil is rich in vitamin C, and as such provides support for the immune system by relieving the effects of colds and flu. It also supports the digestive system by relieving cramp and gas in the intestines. All skin types can benefit from the use of orange oil when used as a skin tonic. Orange oil should always be diluted in a carrier oil.

Precautions: Considered safe

Blends With:

Bergamot	Clary Sage	Clove	Frankincense
Geranium	Ginger	Grapefruit	Jasmine
Lavender	Lemon	Mandarin	Rose
Sandalwood	Ylang Ylang		

Used For:
Digestive System Support
Immune System Support
Good Skin Tonic for all Skin Types

Oregano

Latin Name: *Origanum vulgare*

Note: Middle

Odor Intensity: Medium

Parts Used: Leaves

Extracted By: Steam Distillation

Comes From: Greece, Italy, Mexico, Spain, Turkey, United States

Dilution: Dilute as desired. Can be used topically, diffused or directly inhaled.

Description:

Provides support for the respiratory system for colds and flu. Oregano is also an excellent pain reliever and as such, is used to treat arthritis, rheumatism and muscle strains.

Precautions: Do not use if pregnant. May cause skin irritation if used undiluted. Before diffusing, blend with a mild essential oil such as lavender. Diffused oregano used in excess can cause irritation to the throat and eyes.

Blends With:

Bergamot	Chamomile	Eucalyptus	Geranium	Lavender
Lemon	Pine	Rose	Sandalwood	Tea Tree
Thyme				

Used For:

Respiratory System Support
Arthritis
Rheumatism
Muscle Strains

Patchouli

Latin Name: *Pogostemon cablin*

Note: Base

Odor Intensity: High

Parts Used: Leaves

Extracted By: Steam Distillation

Comes From: China, India, Indonesia, Japan, Madagascar, Malaysia, Philippines, United States

Dilution: Dilute as desired. Can be used topically, diffused or directly inhaled.

Description:

Patchouli is best known as a skin treatment for such conditions as acne and eczema, as it has antifungal properties it is a good treatment for athlete's foot. It is also used for dry and cracked skin. Patchouli provides support for the digestive system in cases of indigestion constipation and colitis.

Precautions: Patchouli should not be ingested as he may react against certain medications.

Blends With:

Bergamot	Chamomile	Cinnamon	Clary Sage
Clove	Coriander	Frankincense	Geranium
Ginger	Grapefruit	Jasmine	Lavender
Lemon	Lemongrass	Mandarin	Myrrh
Neroli	Pine	Rose	Sandalwood
Ylang Ylang			

Used For:
Digestive System Support
Skin Conditions
Athletes Foot

Peppermint

Latin Name: *Mentha piperita*

Note: Top

Odor Intensity: High

Parts Used: Leaves

Extracted By: Steam Distillation

Comes From: Canada, England, France, United States (Michigan)

Dilution: Dilute as desired. Can be used topically, diffused or directly inhaled.

Description:

Peppermint is best known as a support for the digestive system where it is used for indigestion (instead of an antacid), colic, cramps, gas and nausea. In addition, it stimulates the production of bile and provides support for the liver. It is also used for various skin conditions including: acne, dermatitis, itching and sunburn.

Peppermint is used as a memory booster; is excellent in cases of mental fatigue, lack of concentration and memory loss. It can be burnt in an Aromalamp whilst studying for exams to help sharpen the mind and give clarity and understanding to the subject matter.

Precautions: Peppermint may work against homeopathic remedies. Because it stimulates the mind, it might be best not to use it in the evening otherwise sleep patterns may be disturbed. Do not use if pregnant. May cause skin irritation.

Blends With:

Lemon	Eucalyptus	Geranium	Grapefruit	Lavender
Marjoram	Pine	Rosemary	Tea Tree	

Used For:
Digestive System Support
Skin Conditions
Memory Booster

Pine

Latin Name: *Pinus sylvestris*

Note: Middle

Odor Intensity: Medium

Parts Used: Needles

Extracted By: Steam Distillation

Comes From: Finland, Norway, Northern Russia

Dilution: Dilute as desired. Can be used topically, diffused or directly inhaled.

Description:

Pinus sylvestris (Scotch Pine) is native to northern latitudes and is said to be the only European pine to have survived the ice age. Pine supplies strong support for the respiratory system. It kills bacteria and is used for cough, colds, flu, bronchitis and asthma as well as lung infections.

When diluted pine essential oil is added to the bath it will provide relief for cases of arthritis, rheumatism, gout, poor circulation, muscle aches, fatigue and nervous exhaustion. Pine essential oil also supports the immune system in cases of cystitis and other urinary tract infections.

Precautions: Always dilute this oil. May cause skin irritation. Do not use large quantities in the bath. Prostate cancer sufferers should not use Pine.

Blends With:

Bergamot	Eucalyptus	Frankincense	Lavender	Lemon
Marjoram	Patchouli	Peppermint	Rosemary	Thyme

Used For:
Supports the Respiratory System
Supports the Nervous System
Supports the Urinary System
Supports the Circulatory System
Arthritis
Rheumatism
Gout

Rose

Latin Name: *Rosa damascena*

Note: Middle

Oder Intensity: Very High

Parts Used: Flowers

Extracted By: Steam Distillation

Comes From: Bulgaria, France Morocco, Tunisia

Dilution: Dilute as desired. Can be used topically, diffused or directly inhaled.

Description:

Rose is a very expensive oil—it takes the petals of approximately 30 roses to make one drop of Rose Essential Oil. Rose supports the female reproductive system. It helps balance hormones, tones the uterus, stimulates and regulates menstrual flow and menstrual loss. For men, it increases sperm production.

For the respiratory system, it is used for asthma, cough, colds and congestion. In addition, it is used as a treatment for cold sores associated with Herpes Simplex Type 1 virus, as well as a treatment for eczema.

For the nervous system, it provides support in cases of depression, anxiety, anger, sadness, nervous tension and insomnia.

Precautions: Not advised during pregnancy. When purchasing, make sure the oil has not been diluted with geranium essential oil.

Blends With:

Bergamot	Chamomile	Clary Sage	Geranium	Jasmine
Lavender	Lemon	Neroli	Patchouli	
Sandalwood	Yang Ylang			

Used For:
The Female Reproductive System
Supports the Respiratory System
Supports the Nervous System

Rosemary

Latin Name: *Rosmarinus officinalis*

Note: Middle

Odor Density: High

Parts Used: Leaves

Extracted By: Steam Distillation

Comes From: Southern France

Dilution: Dilute as desired. Can be used topically, diffused or directly inhaled.

Description:

Rosemary provides excellent support for the circulatory system in cases of poor circulation, slow blood flow to the heart and for irregular menstruation. Rosemary is an excellent detoxifier for the intestines, liver and gall bladder.

As it has astringent properties, rosemary is also used to tighten loose skin. As it is an antibacterial and antiviral, it is used in cases of acne, dermatitis, eczema and athlete's foot.

Rosemary supports the central nervous system and helps stimulate serotonin production which boosts memory, clears mental fatigue and increases concentration.

Precautions: Do not use if pregnant. Do not use if you have high blood pressure or suffer from epilepsy. May be an irritant to sensitive or damaged skin.

Blends With:

Bergamot	Cinnamon	Clary Sage	Eucalyptus
Frankincense	Geranium	Grapefruit	Lavender
Lemon	Mandarin	Marjoram	Oregano
Peppermint	Pine	Tea Tree	Thyme

Used For:

Supports the Circulatory System
Supports the Nervous System
Detoxifier
Skin Problems
Antibacterial
Antiviral

Sandalwood

Latin Name: *Santalum album*

Note: Base

Odor Intensity: Medium

Parts Used: Heartwood

Extracted By: Steam Distillation

Comes From: Australia, India

Dilution: Dilute as desired. Can be used topically, diffused or directly inhaled.

Description:

Sandalwood is an extremely expensive essential oil due to demand outstripping supply. Sandalwood supplies support for the respiratory system in cases of asthma, bronchitis, expelling excess mucus and cough.

Sandalwood also supports the nervous system in cases of anxiety, depression, fear, insomnia and stress. For the urinary system, it is used to treat cystitis; as it possesses antiseptic properties it acts as a cleanser to increase urine flow.

Precautions: Do not overuse. Do not ingest—can react against certain medications

Blends With:

Bergamot	Chamomile	Frankincense	Geranium	Jasmine
Lavender	Lemon	Myrrh	Neroli	Patchouli
Rose	Ylang Ylang			

Used For:
Supports the Respiratory System
Supports the Nervous System
Supports the Urinary System

Tea Tree

Latin Name: *Melaleuca alternifolia*

Note: Top

Odor Intensity: Very High

Parts Used: Leaves

Extracted By: Steam Distillation

Comes From: Australia

Dilution: Dilute as desired with carrier oil. May be diffused, directly inhaled or topically applied

Description:

Tea Tree is a close cousin of the eucalyptus tree, and as such tea tree should always be in your first aid box. It is excellent for treating bacterial and viral infections. It can be used neat on the skin to treat cases of acne, boils, eczema, and warts. It is also used as a treatment for toe nail infections and athlete's foot. It can be added to skin creams to treat skin rashes and sunburn. It can also be put on mosquito bites to reduce swelling.

Tea Tree provides respiratory system support in cases of colds where it can be used as a gargle It can also be used in cases of asthma, sinus infections and cough. It can be put neat on cold sores associated with the Herpes Simples virus type 1.

Precautions: Although it can be applied neat to the skin, it may cause skin irritation in some individuals

Blends With:

Bergamot	Clary Sage	Clove	Geranium	Grapefruit
Lavender	Marjoram	Pine	Rosemary	Thyme
Peppermint				

Used For:

Bacterial and Viral Infections
Skin Conditions
Supports the Respiratory System
Should be in your first aid box
Seems to be a "cure all" for everything

Thyme Linalol

Latin Name: *Thymus Vvlgaris ct. linalol*

Note: Middle

Odor Intensity: Medium

Parts Used: Leaves and Flowering Tops

Extracted By: Steam Distillation

Comes From: France, Greece, Portugal, Spain, United States

Dilution: Dilute as desired with carrier oil. May be used in a diffuser or topically applied

Description:

Thyme provides support for many of the body's systems: it strengthens and tones the circulatory system; aids the digestive system in the digestion process as well as having an antiseptic action and easing gas and bloating.

Thyme supports the nervous system by relieving symptom of anxiety, depression and stress. It helps boost memory and concentration. It supports the production of white blood cells in the immune system. White blood cells help protect the body against foreign invaders and antigens.

Thyme works in the respiratory system in cases of asthma, colds, cough, laryngitis and sore throat; and in the glandular system as a balancer of the glands and to aid in menstrual flow. As Thyme has an antiseptic action, it provides support to the urinary system by increasing urine flow and assisting in cases of cystitis.

Thyme is useful for various skin conditions including acne, eczema, boils, burns and wound healing, in addition to cold sores associated with the Herpes Simplex Type 1 virus. Thyme can be used for arthritis, rheumatism, gout and muscle strains

Precautions: Do not use if pregnant. May cause skin irritation. Do not ingest or use undiluted. Do not use if you have high blood pressure or suffer from epilepsy.

Thyme Linalol (Cont'd)

Blends With:

Bergamot	Clary Sage	Eucalyptus	Geranium
Grapefruit	Lavender	Lemon	Marjoram
Peppermint	Pine	Rosemary	Tea Tree

Used For:

Supports the Circulatory System
Supports the Digestive System
Supports the Glandular System
Supports the Immune System
Supports the Nervous System
Supports the Respiratory System
Supports the Urinary System
Skin Problems

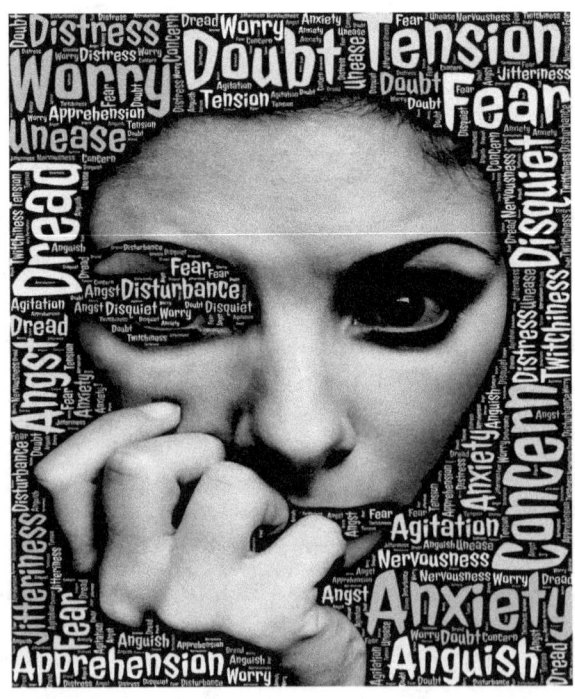

Ylang Ylang

Latin Name: *Cananga odorata*

Note: Base

Odor Intensity: Medium

Parts Used: Flowers

Extracted By: Steam Distillation

Comes From: Indonesia, Madagascar, Philippines, Zanzibar

Dilution: Dilute as desired. Can be used topically, diffused or directly inhaled.

Description:

Ylang Ylang —pronounced "ee long ee long" —meaning "flower of flowers" is grown mainly in Indonesia and Madagascar. The heavily scented flowers which provide this exotic oil are harvested in early morning and are processed straight-away to preserve their odor. Ylang Ylang provides support for the nervous system in cases of panic attack, anxiety, fear and stress. Ylang Ylang is also considered an aphrodisiac and is used for sexual dysfunction due to its calming properties. It is used to treat infections, high blood pressure and to ease the effects of dry skin.

Precautions: Do not use if pregnant. Do not use if you suffer from sleep apnea or low blood pressure. Can be an irritant to sensitive or damaged skin.

Blends With:

Bergamot	Clary Sage	Clove	Jasmine	Lemon
Mandarin	Neroli	Rose	Patchouli	Sandalwood

Used For:

Supports the Nervous System
Sexual Dysfunction
Infections
High Blood Pressure

12. Herbs, Vitamins and Minerals

This book is really about essential oils. But for therapeutic purposes, there is often more to it than just using essential oils. Essential oils are derived from trees and plants—including herbs. When an essential oil is extracted from an herb for example, the essential oil will contains chemicals from the plant it came from. These chemicals perform various functions in the body. As mentioned elsewhere in this book, essential oils are very concentrated—something like 50 times more powerful than if they were left inside the herb plant.

The herb plant does not just contain "oil", but many other compounds such as alkaloids, phytonutrients as well as vitamins and minerals and some of these herb plants also contain antioxidants which help to neutralize free radicals in the body. Also, a herb plant is "balanced" meaning that it may contain natural chemicals to counteract any toxic effects the herb might have. And yes, herbs can be taken along with essential oils. By so doing there is often a synergistic effect where the essential oil helps the herb and the herb helps the essential oil.

Therefore a herbal plant will in all probability have a much milder action in the body, and can often be taken internally without any adverse effects. This is something that cannot be done with an essential oil, which must be diluted first, and then, in all probability, should only be used internally under the supervision of a qualified aromatherapist or doctor. Herbs can be obtained in bulk which you process yourself, as a powder which is inserted into capsules, as a tincture, as an ointment or as a tea.

When we look at all the body systems, they often react to the actions of the individual whose body it is. The body is impartial—it relies on its "owner" to provide the correct amount of nutrients as well as exercise, adequate rest and a wholesome diet to keep it working at optimum efficiency.

Analyzing the modern lifestyle and typical Western diet which is very high in saturated fat, and possibly medications (which produce unwanted side effects) that someone may be taking for a health condition, then there is little wonder that the human body often fails to work at optimum efficiency. This often manifests itself in a compromised digestive and intestinal systems, a weakened immune system and because of everyday stresses and anxiety which often leads to depression—a less than adequate nervous system.

Like all the body systems, the nervous system plays a key role in helping maintain good health. In addition to essential oils such as bergamot, lavender, grapefruit and rose, herbal products as well as vitamin and mineral supplements can also be added. For example, for anxiety and mild to moderate depression St John's Wort is effective. B Complex vitamins and vitamin C are also important. All the B vitamins work together and are best taken in a complex form. You can always top-up with individual B vitamins should you need them. Vitamin C is important too. B vitamins and vitamin C are water soluble and are easily depleted when the body is under stress. For insomnia hops, valerian and passionflower can also be added. Valerian contains natural plant calcium which relaxes the nervous system. None of these herbs are habit forming, and they do not leave you feeling hung-over the following morning either.

And because of an inadequate diet, a lack of exercise and a stressful everyday life, this ultimately can lead to the biggest killer in the Western world—heart disease, which is all part of the circulatory system.

Essential oils will help with all these situations, but at the end of the day, it is up to the individual to have a healthy lifestyle which can comprise a healthy organic diet, which is low in saturated fat, and an adequate intake of vitamins and minerals which because of the lack of minerals in the soil (the human body does not manufacture minerals they have to be obtained from the diet), must be obtained by taking natural (not synthetic) dietary supplements. In addition, omega 3 and 6 essential fatty acids, and possibly a probiotic supplement to maintain friendly bacteria in the gut may need to be added to the diet. Good sources of omega 3 essential fatty acids include oily fish such as salmon, mackerel, tuna and, sardines; krill oil is also another good fish source. If a plant source is preferred then flaxseed oil or blackcurrant oil should be considered. Omega 6 essential fatty acids can be obtained from flax seed oil, evening primrose oil, blackcurrant oil and borage oil. And let's not forget enzymes to help with the breakdown and absorption of nutrients from the food you eat. Vitamins and minerals are the building blocks of proteins, but it is enzymes that do all the work—they make things happen in the body.

And finally, fiber is essential too along with the best quality water you can get (not tap water which is full of chemicals), to help the fiber do its work, and to keep the body hydrated. You need to drink at least eight glasses of water each day—and no, cola drinks don't count. They are full of sugar and chemicals. Fiber keeps everything moving through the colon, in addition to helping soak up toxins in the body. It also helps prevent constipation which is often caused by an inadequate Western diet which is low in fiber content

Having said all of the above, if there is a health problem, it is the body saying "help me". You can use all the essential oils, take all the herbal remedies available, but what is really important is to get to the main reason why there is a health problem, and then deal with it.

The following pages contain a selection of essential oils together with vitamins, minerals and herbal remedies for various health conditions.

With herbs, you may have to do a little experimenting. For example, one person might get a good result from a particular herb, whilst another person might not, but that other person may very likely get a good result from a different herb. Remember, each person is different, and this is reflected in which herbal products will work best for each individual.

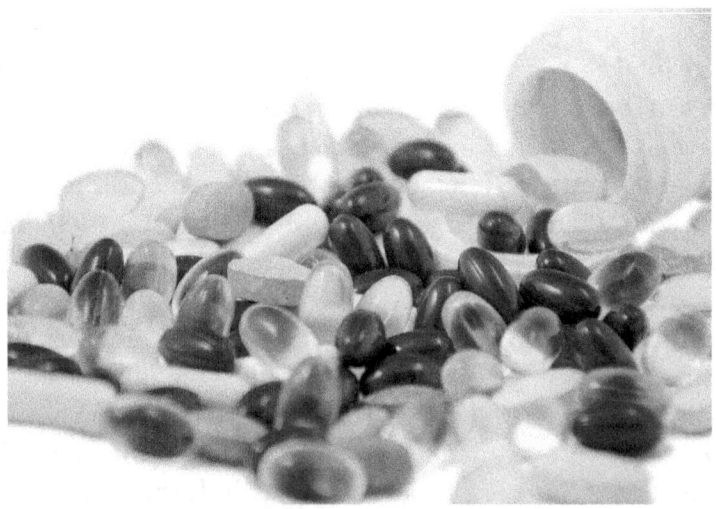

13. Health Conditions

Condition:	**Abdominal Cramps**
Essential Oils:	Clove, Orange, Peppermint, Chamomile
Herbs, Vitamins & Minerals:	Dandelion, Ginger

Condition:	**Acne**
Essential Oils:	Bergamot, Chamomile, Helichrysum, Juniper, Lavender, Lemon, Mandarin, Tea Tree
Herbs, Vitamins & Minerals:	Basil, Burdock, Goldenseal, Oregon Grape

Condition:	**ADD/ADHD**
Essential Oils:	Chamomile, Grapefruit, Lavender, Lemon
Herbs, Vitamins & Minerals:	Calcium/Magnesium, GABA, L-Cysteine, Pantothenic Acid (vitamin B5), Slippery Elm, Vitamin B-Complex

Condition:	**Addiction**
Essential Oils:	Bergamot
Herbs, Vitamins & Minerals:	Kudzu, Lobelia, St. John's Wort

Condition:	**Adrenal Fatigue**
Essential Oils:	Lavender, Pine
Herbs, Vitamins & Minerals:	Bayberry, Licorice, Slippery Elm, Vitamin B-Complex, Vitamin C

Condition:	**Allergies**
Essential Oils:	Chamomile
Herbs, Vitamins & Minerals:	Alfalfa, Burdock, Gymnema Sylvestre, Kudzu, Methyl Sulfonyl Methane (MSM), Yerba Mate

Condition:	**Anemia**
Essential Oils:	Chamomile, Lemon, Peppermint, Thyme
Herbs, Vitamins & Minerals:	Alfalfa, Catnip, Gymnema Sylvestre, Kelp, Maca, Yellow Dock

Condition:	**Aphrodisiac**
Essential Oils:	Clary Sage, Neroli, Orange, Patchouli
Herbs, Vitamins & Minerals:	Ginseng (American, Korean, Siberian)

Condition:	**Anxiety**
Essential Oils:	Bergamot, Chamomile, Clary Sage, Coriander, Frankincense, Hyssop, Juniper, Lavender, Lemon Balm, Neroli, Patchouli, Rose, Sandalwood, Ylang Ylang
Herbs, Vitamins & Minerals:	Calcium/Magnesium, Hops, Kava Kava, Passionflower, Skullcap, St. John's Wort, Valerian, Vitamin B-Complex, Vitamin C

Condition:	**Appetite Stimulant**
Essential Oils:	Clove, Ginger, Rosemary, Oregano
Herbs, Vitamins & Minerals:	Alfalfa

Condition:	**Appetite Suppressant**
Essential Oils:	Bitter Orange
Herbs, Vitamins & Minerals:	Chromium, Garcinia Cambogia, Gymnema Sylvestre, Vitamin B-Complex

Condition:	**Arthritis**
Essential Oils:	Chamomile, Clove, Ginger, Juniper, Oregano, Pine, St. John's Wort, Turmeric
Herbs, Vitamins & Minerals:	Alfalfa, Blue Cohosh, Boneset, Buchu, Buckthorn, Burdock, Capsicum, Chaparral, Echinacea, Fenugreek, Garlic, Gentian, Horsetail, Kelp, Methyl Sulfonyl Methane (MSM), Oatstraw, Olive Leaf, Pau D' Arco, Una De Gato (Cats Claw), White Willow, Yucca

Condition:	**Asthma**
Essential Oils:	Chamomile, Clary Sage, Clove, Frankincense, Ginger, Lavender, Marjoram, Myrrh, Peppermint, Rosemary, Thyme
Herbs, Vitamins & Minerals:	Blue Vervain, Burdock, Elderflower, Elecampane, Garlic, Kelp, Lobelia, Mullein, Wild Cherry, Yerba Mate, Vitamin B-Complex, Vitamin C, Vitamin E

Condition:	**Athlete's Foot**
Essential Oils:	Grapefruit, Lemongrass, Myrrh, Tea Tree
Herbs, Vitamins & Minerals:	Garlic

Condition:	**Bad Breath (See Halitosis)**

Condition:	**Bloating**
Essential Oils:	Juniper, Lemon Balm, Rosemary
Herbs, Vitamins & Minerals:	Buchu, Parsley, Pennyroyal

Condition:	**Blood Pressure, High (See Hypertension)**

Condition:	**Blood Pressure, Low**
Essential Oils:	Eucalyptus, Pine, Rosemary, Thyme
Herbs, Vitamins & Minerals:	Capsicum, Dandelion, Ginkgo Biloba, Licorice, Ginseng (American, Korean, Siberian)

Condition:	**Blood Sugar Levels**
Essential Oils:	Cinnamon
Herbs, Vitamins & Minerals:	Chromium, Black Walnut (Balances), Celery (Reduces), Ginseng (American, Korean, Siberian, Reduces), Gymnema Sylvestre (Balances), Juniper (Balances), Nopal (Balances), Sage (Reduces)

Condition:	**Boils**
Essential Oils:	Bergamot, Chamomile, Eucalyptus, Lavender, Lemon, Myrrh Thyme, Tea Tree
Herbs, Vitamins & Minerals:	Burdock, Chickweed, Chlorophyll, Colloidal Silver, Echinacea, Goldenseal, Garlic, Violet

Condition:	**Bronchitis**
Essential Oils:	Basil, Clove, Frankincense, Ginger, Lemon, Marjoram, Myrrh, Peppermint, Sandalwood, Tea Tree
Herbs, Vitamins & Minerals:	Blue Vervain, Boneset, Burdock, Capsicum, Catnip, Coltsfoot, Elderflower, Elecampane, Fennel, Garlic, Horehound, Lobelia, Marshmallow, Mullein, Saffron, Vitamin C, Wild Cherry, Yerba Santa

Condition:	**Bruises**
Essential Oils:	Chamomile, Helichrysum, Geranium, Lavender
Herbs, Vitamins & Minerals:	Alfalfa, Co-Enzyme Q10 (Co-Q10), Gotu Kola, Vitamin C, Witch Hazel

Condition:	**Burns**
Essential Oils:	Clove, Geranium, Chamomile, Eucalyptus, Lavender, St. John's Wort, Tea Tree
Herbs, Vitamins & Minerals:	Capsicum, Chickweed, Colloidal Silver, Comfrey, Marshmallow, Witch Hazel

Condition:	**Calming**
Essential Oils:	Chamomile, Clary Sage, Lavender
Herbs, Vitamins & Minerals:	Blue Vervain, Passion Flower

Condition:	**Candida (See Yeast Infections)**

Condition:	**Cellulite**
Essential Oils:	Grapefruit, Lemon, Rosemary
Herbs, Vitamins & Minerals:	Lecithin, Kelp, Vitamin C

Condition:	**Chills**
Essential Oils:	Pine, Ginger
Herbs, Vitamins & Minerals:	Boneset

Condition:	**Circulation**
Essential Oils:	Cinnamon, Grapefruit, Rose, Rosemary
Herbs, Vitamins & Minerals:	Bilberry, Blessed Thistle, Butchers Broom, Catnip, Elderflower, Ginkgo Biloba, Gotu Kola, Hawthorn

Condition:	**Cold Sores (Herpes Simplex Type 1 Virus)**
Essential Oils:	Bergamot, Geranium, Lemon Balm, Marjoram, Myrrh, Patchouli, Tea Tree, Thyme
Herbs, Vitamins & Minerals:	Hyssop, Licorice, L-Lysine, Olive Leaf, Vitamin C

Condition:	**Cold**
Essential Oils:	Cinnamon, Clove, Frankincense, Ginger, Grapefruit, Lavender, Lemon, Lemongrass, Myrrh, Oregano, Peppermint, Pine, Tea Tree
Herbs, Vitamins & Minerals:	Basil, Blue Vervain, Boneset, Capsicum, Caraway, Catnip, Colloidal Silver, Echinacea, Elderflower, Garlic, Goldenseal, Hibiscus, Kudzu, Marshmallow, Mullein, Olive Leaf, Sarsaparilla, Wild Cherry, Vitamin C

Condition:	**Colic**
Essential Oils:	Chamomile, Ginger, Lemon Balm
Herbs, Vitamins & Minerals:	Blue Cohosh, Catnip, Fennel

Condition:	**Colitis**
Essential Oils:	Chamomile, Clove, Geranium, Neroli, Peppermint
Herbs, Vitamins & Minerals:	Black Walnut, Psyllium, Una De Gato (Cats Claw)

Condition:	Congestion
Essential Oils:	Ginger, Marjoram, Myrrh, Oregano
Herbs, Vitamins & Minerals:	Blue Vervain, Burdock, Elderflower, Hyssop, Mullein, Yerba Santa

Condition:	**Constipation**
Essential Oils:	Lemon, Orange
Herbs, Vitamins & Minerals:	Aloe Vera, Black Walnut, Boneset, Cascara Sagrada, Chickweed, Gymnema Sylvestre, Magnesium, Oregon Grape, Psyllium, Red Raspberry, Yerba Mate

Condition:	Cough
Essential Oils:	Cinnamon, Clary Sage, Eucalyptus, Frankincense, Ginger, Jasmine, Lemongrass, Marjoram, Myrrh, Pine, Rosemary, Sandalwood, Thyme
Herbs, Vitamins & Minerals:	Basil, Coltsfoot, Garlic, Gymnema Sylvestre, Horehound, Hyssop, Kelp, Lobelia, Marshmallow, Mullein, Pennyroyal, Sarsaparilla, Wild Cherry

Cramp	**Catnip, Coriander, Ginger, Hops, Chamomile, Marjoram, Turmeric**
Cramp, Menstrual	Black Cohosh, Blessed Thistle, Caraway, Catnip, Dandelion, White Willow
Cramp, Muscle	Blue Cohosh, Catnip

Condition:	**Cuts and Scrapes**
Essential Oils:	Eucalyptus, St. John's Wort
Herbs, Vitamins & Minerals:	Marshmallow, Witch Hazel, Yarrow

Condition:	**Cystitis**
Essential Oils:	Bergamot, Clove, Lavender, Sandalwood, Tea Tree
Herbs, Vitamins & Minerals:	Buchu, Corn Silk, Cranberry, Horsetail, Hydrangea, Marshmallow, Parsley, Uva Ursi

Condition:	**Dandruff**
Essential Oils:	Eucalyptus, Lavender, Peppermint, Rosemary, Sage, Thyme
Herbs, Vitamins & Minerals:	Burdock, Evening Primrose Oil, Flaxseed Oil, Horsetail, Kelp, Vitamin B-Complex

Condition:	**Decongestant**
Essential Oils:	Patchouli, Thyme
Herbs, Vitamins & Minerals:	Hyssop, Pennyroyal, Yerba Santa

Condition:	**Depression**
Essential Oils:	Bergamot, Clary Sage, Lemon Balm, Frankincense, Geranium, Grapefruit, Jasmine, Lavender, Lemon, Neroli, Orange, Patchouli, Peppermint, Rose, Sandalwood, Thyme, Ylang Ylang
Herbs, Vitamins & Minerals:	Maca, Oatstraw, St John's Wort, Valerian, Yohimbe

Condition:	**Detox**
Essential Oils:	Bergamot, Catnip, Coriander, Ginger, Lemon, Grapefruit, Helichrysum
Herbs, Vitamins & Minerals:	Activated Charcoal, Alfalfa, Bentonite Clay, Chlorophyll, Dandelion, Lecithin, SAMe, Vitamin B-Complex, Vitamin C

Condition:	**Diabetes** (See Blood Sugar Levels)

Condition:	**Diarrhea**
Essential Oils:	Cilantro, Ginger, Neroli
Herbs, Vitamins & Minerals:	Bayberry, Bentonite Clay, Blackberry, Catnip, Marshmallow, Mullein, Oregon Grape, Red Raspberry, Uva Ursi, Witch Hazel

Condition:	**Digestive Problems**
Essential Oils:	Cilantro, Cinnamon, Dill, Ginger, Juniper, Lemon Balm, Marjoram, Myrrh, Neroli: Oregano, Peppermint, Rosemary, Tarragon, Thyme, Turmeric
Herbs, Vitamins & Minerals:	Alfalfa, Blessed Thistle, Capsicum, Caraway, Catnip. Fennel, Gentian, Goldenseal, Hops, Nopal, Parsley, Pau D'Arco, Pennyroyal, Wild Cherry

Condition:	**Eczema**
Essential Oils:	Bergamot, Geranium, Chamomile, Juniper, Lemon Balm, Sandalwood
Herbs, Vitamins & Minerals:	Burdock, Goldenseal, Horehound, Kelp, Oregon Grape, Pau D'Arco

Condition:	**Edema** (See Water Retention)

Condition:	**Fatigue**
Essential Oils:	Lemongrass, Peppermint, Pine, Thyme
Herbs, Vitamins & Minerals:	Alfalfa, Hawthorn, Kelp

Condition:	**Fever**
Essential Oils:	Pine, Ginger
Herbs, Vitamins & Minerals:	Alfalfa, Bayberry, Blessed Thistle, Boneset, Buckthorn, Catnip, Elderflower, Hyssop, Lobelia, Olive Leaf, Parsley, Sage, Sarsaparilla, White Willow

Condition:	**Flu**
Essential Oils:	Eucalyptus, Ginger, Marjoram, Oregano, Tea Tree
Herbs, Vitamins & Minerals:	Basil, Bayberry, Boneset, Catnip, Colloidal Silver, Echinacea, Elderflower, Garlic, Goldenseal, Hibiscus, Kudzu, L-Lysine, Marshmallow, Olive Leaf, Pau D'Arco

Condition:	**Fungal Infections**
Essential Oils:	Geranium, Grapefruit, Lemon, Mandarin, Myrrh, Patchouli, Tea Tree, Thyme
Herbs, Vitamins & Minerals:	Acidophilus, Caprylic Acid, Colloidal Silver, Garlic, Kelp, Pau D'Arco, Vitamin C

Condition:	**Gas**
Essential Oils:	Lemon Balm
Herbs, Vitamins & Minerals:	Barberry, Caraway, Fennel, Parsley, Pennyroyal, Slippery Elm, Yucca

Condition:	**Gout**
Essential Oils:	Basil, Juniper
Herbs, Vitamins & Minerals:	Buckthorn, Burdock, Horsetail, Sarsaparilla

Condition:	**Hair Loss**
Essential Oils:	Clary Sage, Lavender, Rosemary Thyme
Herbs, Vitamins & Minerals:	Alfalfa, Evening Primrose Oil, Flax Seed Oil, Horsetail, Vitamin B-Complex, Vitamin B6

Condition:	**Halitosis**
Essential Oils:	Bergamot, Clove, Myrrh, Peppermint, Rosemary
Herbs, Vitamins & Minerals:	Alfalfa, Chaparral, Chlorophyll, L-Cysteine, Parsley, SAMe

Condition:	**Headache**
Essential Oils:	Eucalyptus, Tea Tree, Lavender, Lemongrass, Oregano, Peppermint, Rosemary, St. John's Wort
Herbs, Vitamins & Minerals:	Basil, Black Cohosh, Blessed Thistle, Blue Vervain, Catnip, Celery Dong Quai, Saffron, White Willow

Condition:	**Heart Palpitations**
Essential Oils:	Clary Sage, Neroli
Herbs, Vitamins & Minerals:	Black Cohosh

Condition:	**Hemorrhoids**
Essential Oils:	Chamomile, Geranium, Myrrh, Pine
Herbs, Vitamins & Minerals:	Blackberry, Buckthorn, Butchers Broom, Cascara Sagrada, Garlic, Horsetail, Mullein, Nettle, Pau D'Arco, Psyllium, Shepherds Purse, Slippery Elm, St. John's Wort, Vitamin C, Witch Hazel

Condition:	**Herpes Simplex Virus (Type 1 & 11) Cold Sores, Blisters**
Essential Oils:	Geranium, Lemon Balm, Marjoram
Herbs, Vitamins & Minerals:	Horehound, Hyssop, Licorice, Olive Leaf

Condition:	**Hiccups**
Essential Oils:	Dill, Fennel, Tarragon
Herbs, Vitamins & Minerals:	Blue Cohosh

Condition:	**Hormone Balance**
Essential Oils:	Clary Sage, Geranium, Rose, Sage
Herbs, Vitamins & Minerals:	Borage Oil, Evening Primrose Oil, Flaxseed Oil, Omega-3 EPA

Condition:	**Hot Flashes**
Essential Oils:	Clary Sage, Geranium, Lavender, Pine
Herbs, Vitamins & Minerals:	Alfalfa, Barberry, Calcium/Magnesium, Capsicum, Celery, Co-Enzyme Q10 (Co-Q10), Dandelion, Dong Quai, Flaxseed Oil, Garlic, L-Glutamine, Hibiscus, Kelp, Kudzu, Lecithin, Nettle, Omega-3 EPA, Parsley, Passionflower, Pau D'Arco, Vitamin B-Complex, Vitamin E

Condition:	**Immune System Support**
Essential Oils:	Chamomile, Eucalyptus, Lemon, Lime, Orange
Herbs, Vitamins & Minerals:	Barberry, Boneset, Echinacea, Garlic, Ginseng (American, Korean, Siberian), Maca, Olive Leaf, Pau D'Arco, Una De Gato (Cats Claw)

Condition:	**Impotence**
Essential Oils:	Bergamot, Jasmine, Rose, Sandalwood
Herbs, Vitamins & Minerals:	Ginkgo Biloba, Maca, Vitamin B-Complex, Yohimbe, Zinc

Condition:	**Indigestion**
Essential Oils:	Ginger, Peppermint
Herbs, Vitamins & Minerals:	Barberry, Boneset, Hops, Hyssop, Parsley

Condition:	**Infection**
Essential Oils:	Bergamot, Chamomile, Cilantro, Eucalyptus, Lemon, Lime, Tea Tree, Thyme
Herbs, Vitamins & Minerals:	Alfalfa, Barberry, Basil, Boneset, Buchu, Burdock, Cranberry, Dandelion, Echinacea, Fenugreek Garlic, Gentian, Goldenseal, Hyssop, Juniper, Kelp, Olive Leaf, Oregon Grape, Parsley, Pau D'Arco, Uva Ursi

Condition:	Inflammation
Essential Oils:	Bergamot, Chamomile, Cinnamon, Clary Sage, Eucalyptus, Lavender, Lemongrass, Turmeric
Herbs, Vitamins & Minerals:	Blue Cohosh, Capsicum, Chaparral, Chickweed, Elderflower, Gentian, Horsetail, Hyssop, Hydrangea, Licorice, Marshmallow, Olive Leaf, Pau D'Arco, Una De Gato (Cats Claw), Uva Ursi, White Willow, Witch Hazel, Yucca

Condition:	Insect Repellent
Essential Oils:	Lemon Balm, Tea Tree
Herbs, Vitamins & Minerals:	Basil, Pennyroyal

Condition:	**Insomnia**
Essential Oils:	Chamomile, Lavender, Lemon Balm, Marjoram, Neroli, Sandalwood
Herbs, Vitamins & Minerals:	Basil, Calcium/Magnesium, Blue Vervain, Celery, Hops, Kava Kava, Passionflower, Skullcap, Valerian

Condition:	**Irritable Bowel Syndrome**
Essential Oils:	Chamomile, Peppermint
Herbs, Vitamins & Minerals:	Acidophilus, Alfalfa, Aloe Vera, Alpha Lipoic Acid, Calcium/Magnesium, L-Glutamine, Slippery Elm, Valerian, Vitamin B-Complex

Condition:	**Itching**
Essential Oils:	Chamomile, Lavender, Sandalwood
Herbs, Vitamins & Minerals:	Buckthorn

Condition:	**Jet Lag**
Essential Oils:	Chamomile, Clary Sage, Lavender, Geranium, Marjoram, Peppermint
Herbs, Vitamins & Minerals:	Hops, Melatonin, Passionflower, Valerian

Condition:	**Kidney Problems**
Essential Oils:	Celery, Juniper
Herbs, Vitamins & Minerals:	Bilberry, Black Cohosh, Buchu, Burdock, Capsicum, Hawthorn, Horsetail, Parsley, Saffron

Condition:	**Laryngitis**
Essential Oils:	Jasmine, Thyme
Herbs, Vitamins & Minerals:	Lobelia

Condition:	**Liver Tonic**
Essential Oils:	Chamomile, Geranium, Grapefruit, Helichrysum
Herbs, Vitamins & Minerals:	Alfalfa, Barberry, Bayberry, Milk Thistle, Nopal, Oregon Grape, Saffron, Yellow Dock, Yucca

Condition:	**Lymphatic System**
Essential Oils:	Grapefruit, Lemon, Sandalwood
Herbs, Vitamins & Minerals:	Burdock, Yellow Dock

Condition:	**Menopause**
Essential Oils:	Clary Sage, Geranium, Chamomile, Sage
Herbs, Vitamins & Minerals:	Black Cohosh, Dong Quai, Red Clover

Condition:	**Menstrual Problems**
Essential Oils:	Clary Sage, Geranium, Chamomile, Marjoram, Myrrh, Rose, Sage
Herbs, Vitamins & Minerals:	Black Cohosh, Blessed Thistle

Condition:	Migraine
Essential Oils:	Chamomile, Lemon, Rosemary
Herbs, Vitamins & Minerals:	Black Cohosh, Dong Quai

Condition:	**Morning Sickness**
Essential Oils:	Ginger
Herbs, Vitamins & Minerals:	Catnip

Condition:	**Mouth Ulcers**
Essential Oils:	Clove, Myrrh, Tea Tree
Herbs, Vitamins & Minerals:	Aloe Vera, Colloidal Silver

Condition:	Muscle Aches And Pains
Essential Oils:	Chamomile, Cinnamon, Eucalyptus, Ginger, Grapefruit, Helichrysum, Jasmine, Lavender, Oregano, Pine, St. John's Wort, Turmeric
Herbs, Vitamins & Minerals:	Buchu, Calcium/Magnesium

Condition:	Muscle Cramps & Spasms
Essential Oils:	Catnip
Herbs, Vitamins & Minerals:	Blue Cohosh, Horsetail, Valerian

Condition:	Nausea (Also See Vomiting)
Essential Oils:	Ginger, Peppermint, Turmeric
Herbs, Vitamins & Minerals:	Wild Yam

Condition:	**Nervous Tension**
Essential Oils:	Chamomile, Jasmine, Lavender, Marjoram, Neroli, Rose, Sandalwood, Ylang Ylang
Herbs, Vitamins & Minerals:	Hops, St. John's Wort, Valerian,

Condition:	**Neuralgia**
Essential Oils:	Chamomile, Clove, Helichrysum, Geranium, Lavender, Peppermint
Herbs, Vitamins & Minerals:	Blue Cohosh, Calcium/Magnesium, Celery, Hops, Methyl Sulfonyl Methane (MSM), Potassium, Valerian, Vitamin B-Complex

Condition:	**Night Sweats**
Essential Oils:	Clary Sage
Herbs, Vitamins & Minerals:	Black Cohosh

Condition:	Pain Relief
Essential Oils:	Chamomile, Clove, Peppermint, Rose, Tea Tree
Herbs, Vitamins & Minerals:	Hops, Valerian

Condition:	Panic Attacks
Essential Oils:	Ylang Ylang
Herbs, Vitamins & Minerals:	Kava Kava, Valerian

Condition:	**Premenstrual Syndrome (PMS)**
Essential Oils:	Chamomile, Clary Sage, Geranium, Juniper, Lavender, Marjoram, Neroli
Herbs, Vitamins & Minerals:	Dandelion, Dong Quai, Magnesium

Condition:	**Prostate**
Essential Oils:	Juniper, Myrrh
Herbs, Vitamins & Minerals:	Buchu Goldenseal, Gotu Kola, Hydrangea, Kelp, Nettle, Pumpkin, Saw Palmetto

Condition:	Parasites
Essential Oils:	Bergamot, Chamomile, Clove, Ginger, Oregano, Rosemary, Tea Tree, Thyme **Ascaris & Oxyuris:** Eucalyptus, Chamomile; **Hookworm:** Clove, Thyme; **Tapeworm:** Thyme; **Roundworm:** Chamomile, Eucalyptus, Thyme; **Pinworm/Threadworm:** Chamomile, Eucalyptus, Lemon, Thyme
Herbs, Vitamins & Minerals:	Anamu, Artemesia, Basil, Black Walnut, Buckthorn, Elecampane, Garlic, Hyssop, Pumpkin, Olive Leaf, Oregon Grape,

Condition:	**Psoriasis**
Essential Oils:	Bergamot, Chamomile, Lavender, Helichrysum
Herbs, Vitamins & Minerals:	Burdock, Flaxseed Oil, Gotu Kola, Kelp, Omega-3 EPA, Oregon Grape, Pau D'Arco

Condition:	**Rashes**
Essential Oils:	Chamomile
Herbs, Vitamins & Minerals:	Goldenseal

Condition:	**Respiratory Infections**
Essential Oils:	Eucalyptus, Ginger
Herbs, Vitamins & Minerals:	Basil, Coltsfoot, Comfrey, Elderflower, Fenugreek, Hibiscus, Lobelia, Mullein, Olive Leaf

Condition:	**Rheumatism**
Essential Oils:	Cinnamon, Frankincense, Oregano, Pine, Turmeric
Herbs, Vitamins & Minerals:	Boneset, Horsetail, Nettle

Condition:	**Ringworm**
Essential Oils:	Eucalyptus, Geranium, Grapefruit, Lemon, Myrrh, Patchouli, Tea Tree
Herbs, Vitamins & Minerals:	Black Walnut

Condition:	**Sexual Dysfunction: (See Impotence)**

Condition:	Shingles (Herpes Zoster Virus)
Essential Oils:	Geranium
Herbs, Vitamins & Minerals:	Horehound (Applied Topically)

Condition:	**Sinusitis**
Essential Oils:	Clove, Eucalyptus, Lavender, Lemon, Oregano, Peppermint, Pine, Tea Tree, Thyme
Herbs, Vitamins & Minerals:	Capsicum, Fenugreek, Garlic

Condition:	**Skin Conditions**
Essential Oils:	Bergamot, Chamomile, Geranium, Lavender, Mandarin, Patchouli
Herbs, Vitamins & Minerals:	Chickweed (Apply Externally), Gotu Kola, Horehound (Apply Externally), Kelp, Yellow Dock (Apply Externally)

Condition:	**Sore Throat**
Essential Oils:	Chamomile, Ginger, Myrrh, Oregano, Thyme
Herbs, Vitamins & Minerals:	Colloidal Silver, Bayberry, Blue Cohosh, Capsicum, Elderflower, Fenugreek, Marshmallow, Mullein, Sage, Violet, Witch Hazel

Condition:	**Stress**
Essential Oils:	Bergamot, Chamomile, Grapefruit, Hops, Lavender, Lemongrass, Mandarin, Patchouli, Peppermint, Rose, Rosemary, Sandalwood, Ylang Ylang
Herbs, Vitamins & Minerals:	Calcium/Magnesium, Ginseng (American, Korean, Siberian), Hops, Juniper, Licorice Passion Flower, Pumpkin, St. John's Wort, Valerian, Vitamin B-Complex, Vitamin C

Condition:	**Sunburn**
Essential Oils:	Lavender
Herbs, Vitamins & Minerals:	Aloe Vera, St. John's Wort

Condition:	**Teething Pain**
Essential Oils:	Chamomile
Herbs, Vitamins & Minerals:	Aloe Vera, Colloidal Silver

Condition:	**Tonsillitis**
Essential Oils:	Oregano
Herbs, Vitamins & Minerals:	Black Walnut

Condition:	**Tension**
Essential Oils:	Clary Sage, Coriander, Frankincense, Grapefruit, Jasmine, Lavender, Marjoram
Herbs, Vitamins & Minerals:	Calcium/Magnesium, Hops, Kava Kava, Passion Flower, Valerian, Vitamin B-Complex, Vitamin C

Condition:	**Tooth Ache**
Essential Oils:	Chamomile, Clove
Herbs, Vitamins & Minerals:	White Willow

Condition:	**Ulcer**
Essential Oils:	Bergamot, Chamomile, Cinnamon, Myrrh, Rose, Sage
Herbs, Vitamins & Minerals:	Chickweed, Gotu Kola, Kelp, Licorice, Papaya, Pau D'Arco, Una De Gato (Cats Claw), Violet

Condition:	**Urinary Tract Infection**
Essential Oils:	Bergamot
Herbs, Vitamins & Minerals:	Buchu, Cranberry, Horsetail, Hydrangea, Juniper, Oregon Grape, Parsley, Uva Ursi

Condition:	**Vaginal Infection**
Essential Oils:	Eucalyptus
Herbs, Vitamins & Minerals:	Caprylic Acid

Condition:	**Varicose Veins**
Essential Oils:	Bergamot, Frankincense, Geranium, Lemon, Rose
Herbs, Vitamins & Minerals:	Bilberry, Butchers Broom, Capsicum, Co-Enzyme Q10 (Co-Q10), Garlic, Ginkgo Biloba, Gotu Kola, Lecithin, Psyllium, Vitamin C, Vitamin E

Condition:	**Viral Infection**
Essential Oils:	Cinnamon, Eucalyptus, Lemon Balm, Marjoram
Herbs, Vitamins & Minerals:	Horehound (Apply Topically), Hyssop, Licorice, Olive Leaf, St John's Wort, Una De Gato (Cats Claw)

Condition:	**Vomiting (Also See Nausea)**
Essential Oils:	Lemon Balm
Herbs, Vitamins & Minerals::	Catnip

Condition:	**Warts**
Essential Oils:	Cinnamon, Helichrysum
Herbs, Vitamins & Minerals:	Buckthorn, Colloidal Silver

Condition:	**Water Retention (Also See Edema)**
Essential Oils:	Grapefruit, Juniper
Herbs, Vitamins & Minerals:	Buchu, Hydrangea, Hyssop

Condition:	**Weight Loss**
Essential Oils:	Bitter Orange, Grapefruit
Herbs, Vitamins & Minerals:	Celery, Dandelion, Garcinia Cambogia, Nopal, Yerba Mate, Yohimbe

Condition:	**Wounds**
Essential Oils:	Bergamot, Chamomile, Eucalyptus, Helichrysum, Myrrh, Rose, Tea Tree, Thyme
Herbs, Vitamins & Minerals:	Blackberry, Black Walnut, Burdock, Colloidal Silver, Fenugreek, Goldenseal, Hyssop, Marshmallow, Pau D'Arco, Shepherds Purse, St John's Wort, Uva Ursi

Condition:	**Yeast Infection**
Essential Oils:	Bergamot, Eucalyptus, Ginger, Lavender, Oregano, Patchouli, Peppermint, Rosemary Tea Tree, Thyme
Herbs, Vitamins & Minerals:	Acidophilus, Caprylic Acid, Flaxseed Oil, Garlic, Olive Leaf, Omega-3 EPA, Pau D'Arco, Vitamin B-Complex, Vitamin C

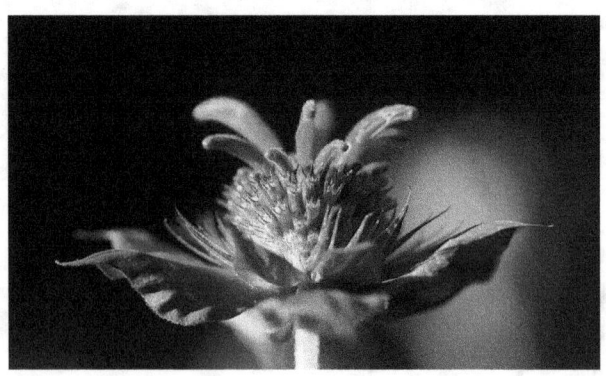

14. Sample Essential Oil Recipes

Essential oils can be extremely useful to treat conditions of the nervous system. Remember to store all essential oils in a dark amber or dark blue colored bottle. Also, use a glass eye dropper to measure out the correct number of drops—do not use plastic. Patch test all essential oil blends on a small area of skin to make sure they do not cause an allergic reaction. Store all essential oils in a cool, dark place and away from children and pets.

Here are two recipes that can be used for relaxation and sexual stimulation:

Recipe For Relaxation

1 ounce of carrier oil
5 drops of Lavender
3 drops of Sandalwood

As sandalwood is expensive, you can substitute rose or mandarin if you wish.

It is important to set the mood to get the maximum benefit from a relaxation session. Light a few candles and play some soothing music. Massage your partner with warmed massage oil beginning at the base of the neck and working your way down the back. Rub shoulders and muscles throughout the back and allow the magic of the healing oils to get to work.

Recipe For Sexual Stimulation

1 ounce of carrier oil
6 drops of Jasmine
2 drops of Bergamot

Jasmine is an effective way to promote confidence and stimulation. To set the mood, use the above recipe to give your partner a massage. This will help him or her relax and enjoy lovemaking. Speak softly and lovingly to your partner as you use this special blend.

Pain Relief

A deep tissue massage is one way to relieve pain that is caused by physical activity. In addition to pain relief, you can use this recipe to sooth aching feet by rubbing firmly with your thumbs into the souls of your feet as well as the heels. This massage treatment is especially good for relieving arthritic joint pain.

Massage Recipe For Pain Relief

I ounce of carrier oil
4 drops of Chamomile
4 drops of Tea Tree

Bath Oil

Aromatherapy bath oils can be used in a similar way to massage oils. The concept is basically the same—you take a warm and relaxing bath with water that contains about a quarter of a cup of aromatherapy bath oil. The oils penetrate the skin and this is when they do their work.

Why not make enough bath oil to last for several baths? You can do this by doubling up on the quantities. Another way of doing it is to add 10 drops of essential oils to 1 ounce of carrier oil. Essential oil blends will last for about one year if stored in a cool dark place, in amber or bark blue bottles and with the top screwed on tight.

Here is a recipe for a relaxing bath oil:

2 ounces of carrier oil
12 drops of Lavender
6 drops of Rose
2 drops of Tea Tree

Make sure you blend the oils properly and only use about a quarter of a cup of oil in the bath. Lavender, rose and tea tree are all very pleasant and soothing and will provide a very relaxing bath.

For menstrual cramps or any instances of stomach pain, try the following:

Pain Relief Bath Oil Recipe

2 ounces of carrier oil
10 drops of Rose
4 drops of Peppermint
6 drops of Chamomile

Soaking in a warm tub is one way to relieve stomach cramps caused either by stress or your menstrual cycle.

Bath Salts

Let's now have a look at bath salts to put in your bath water. You can use Epsom salts or Dead Sea salts to do this. You can buy both online. Epsom salts can be bought from your local drug store. Here's how to make some really great smelling bath salts:

Combine three cups of salts, one tablespoon of carrier oil and 20 drops of essential oil (use the bath oil recipe essential oil suggestions on the previous page) in a bowl—remember do not use a plastic bowl! Mix using a metal fork or spoon (or a wooden spoon) until everything is well mixed. Put in a glass jar with a tight fitting lid. Store in a dark cool place away from children and pets.

To use, sprinkle half a cup of the salts into the bath tub under warm running water and wait for the salts to dissolve before stepping into the bath.

Bath salts are very popular because they are very easy to store and there is a minimal risk of spillage.

If you want to make exotic looking bath salts, then, you can use Hawaiian Red Sea Salt which has a natural salmon color. Another way, you can add the Hawaiian Sea Salt to Epsom salts if you prefer. Do not use vegetable oil food dyes to color the salts as these oils can turn the skin the same color as the vegetable oil food dye in the bath. You will then have the chore of doing several baths to wash the color out of the skin.

Here is another recipe using bath salts that is ideal for relaxation and to help you sleep:

Calming Bath Salts Recipe

3 cups of Epsom salts
1 tablespoon carrier oil
10 drops of Chamomile
5 drops of Lavender
4 drops of Tea Tree
1 drop of Lemon

You will enjoy taking a bath using aromatherapy bath salts that can ease aching joints and, ease tension, relieve cramps and be relaxing before going to bed. Beware when you start making bath oils and bath salts—it can become very addictive and you will soon be hooked. Very likely you will start to give them away as gifts to friends and family who can also benefit from your healthful creations.

Acne

When using aromatherapy and essential oils to treat acne, it is best to use light carrier oil rather than heavy oil—there are some light vegetable oils available which are ideal for the purpose. The essential oils that encourage acne healing include lavender, (which cures just about everything), bergamot and tea tree.

Lavender is one of the few essential oils that is safe to use directly on your skin (provided that you do not have a sensitive skin—patch test first), you can use this essential oil alone and put a drop on the affected area. Alternatively you can use this recipe:

Acne Treatment Recipe

1 ounce of carrier oil
15 drops of Lavender
4 drops of Bergamot
2 drops of Lemon

As mentioned elsewhere in this book, bergamot is photo sensitive, meaning that you should not go out in sunlight for 12 hours after using it. Here is a good way to use it. Use the recipe at night before going to bed, then in the morning rinse it off before going outside. You can create a topical ointment by adding your essential oils to a fragrance free cream or aloe vera gel, then apply as necessary.

Treating acne also involve healing from the inside. Some research suggests that stress can be a trigger for an acne breakout. You can therefore eliminate stress and create a relaxing environment by using an essential oil bath or massage oils.

In addition the following vitamins, minerals and herbal supplements are helpful for treating a stress condition: calcium/magnesium, vitamin D, ginseng (American, Korean, Siberian), hops, juniper, licorice passionflower, pumpkin, St. John's wort, valerian, vitamin B-Complex, vitamin C.

Calcium and magnesium are calming to the nervous system and are best taken in the evening before going to bed. Vitamin D is often thought of as the "sunshine vitamin" as it is synthesized in the body through exposure to sunlight. The body needs this vitamin for the uptake of calcium and magnesium. Ginseng provides energy; licorice supports the adrenal glands; valerian is a source of natural plant calcium, and works with hops and passionflower to create calm, promote sleep in cases of insomnia and settle an overworked mind. Vitamin B-Complex and vitamin C are water soluble vitamins which are easily depleted when the body is under stress.

Diffusing Essential Oils

Using a diffusion method to disperse essential oils in a room is ideal for anyone who has skin sensitivity to the essential oils. In addition, the scent from the oils can also benefit anyone else who is in the room at the same time.

When essential oils are inhaled into the lungs, they cause the same reaction as when they are applied to the skin. All that needs to be done is to pour the essential oil or oil blend into a diffuser and by breathing in the scent of the oil; you will achieve a good health benefit. As mentioned elsewhere in this book, diffusers can be either candle powered or powered by electricity.

When using essential oils as a mood enhancer in a diffuser, there is no need to dilute the essential oils. You can use any essential oils that you like, or use a combination of essential oils, to create the mood you want. Here are some ways you can use essential oils in a variety of different diffusers:

Mood Enhancer Recipe

5 drops of Orange
5 drops of Jasmine

Do not use the scents that are sold in craft stores as they are usually not true essential oils but synthetic scents.

Put your essential oil selection into the diffuser, light the candle underneath or plug into the electrical outlet and let the scent fill the room.

Romantic Mood Enhancer Recipe

In a light ring put either 2 drops of Patchouli, Jasmine or Ylang Ylang. The heat from the light bulb will heat the oil and the scent will spread throughout the room. All of these essential oils are potent aphrodisiacs.

Relaxing Diffusion Recipe

Purchase an electric diffuser that is used to heat potpourri oil and put it on the dresser in your room. Add the following to the diffuser:

10 drops of Chamomile
2 drops of Vanilla
2 drops of Lavender

The scent created by this recipe is really relaxing and calming as it takes over the room.

Scent has a lot to do with how we feel. The scent from the essential oils sends a signal to the brain which releases endorphins. It is not difficult to put yourself in a better mood by the use of scent, which is the basic concept of aromatherapy.

When we discuss aromatherapy we are explaining the use of essential oils to promote healing. However, the scent of the essential oils is a vital part of the healing powers used in this alternative medicine approach. Even when you are using essential oils topically, you are still breathing in the scent and getting the full effect of the true treatment.

You do not just have to use aromatherapy and essential oils to heal. You can just use the essential oils to make your home smell nice for your own enjoyment. As they are very concentrated, essential oils can be useful in homes where smokers or pets reside.

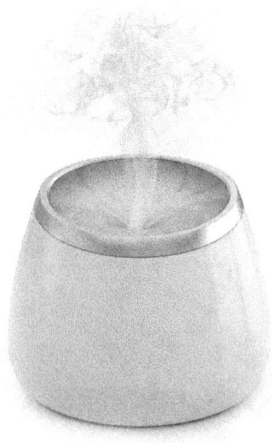

15. Essential Oils Basic Care Kit

Aromatherapy is not difficult to do; however, it is a good idea to put together a basic care kit to get you started. The following are some suggestions for you to consider.

Lavender

Lavender essential oil is so versatile. Here are some suggestions. You can search for many more on the Internet.

- **Calming** – You can put a few drops of lavender oil on a cotton ball and inhale the scent to create calmness. You can discretely use it in crowded places, in your car, or office. You can also put it in a diffuser and spritz the air. It can also be added to lotions to rub on your hands and arms, inhaling the scent as you do to enhance calmness. It will also help you get a good night's sleep.

- **Insect Bites, Minor Cuts & Burns, Skin Issues, Cold Sores & Dandruff** – Putting a few drops of lavender oil into a carrier oil then rubbing it into your skin, scalp or on an insect bite or skin irritation can help soothe the skin and heal the problem.

- **Nausea & Motion Sickness** – Put a couple drops of lavender oil behind your ears for motion sickness and nausea.

- **Nosebleeds** – Make a compress with a few drops of lavender oil on a tissue or cloth and then press it under the base of the nose to help stop the bleeding.

- **In Food** – Lavender oil is one of the few essential oils that you can ingest without medical supervision. It is excellent in recipes and iced tea. It can help reduce the effects of allergies.

Lavender is a truly versatile essential oil with many uses. Most people love the smell of lavender so it can be safely used to help an entire household relax. Why not grow some lavender in your garden? It is very easy to cultivate, requiring almost no watering or care after you plant it.

Tea Tree

Tea Tree oil is native to Australia. It can be used to treat many health conditions from acne to sunburn if you know how.

- **Acne** – Add a couple of drops of tea tree oil to an unscented lotion and then apply to the affected area every night to help the healing process.

- **Athlete's Foot** – Add some tea tree oil to a bowl of warm water to soak your feet in. In addition to helping cure this fungal infection, it can also be used to treat other yeast related infections as well.

- **Antiseptic** – Add to a lotion for use on cuts, burns and other skin problems. It kills germs and prevents infection.

- **Chest Congestion** – Put some tea tree oil into a vaporizer to help loosen chest congestion.

Tea tree oil can also be used to treat headaches, colds and even lice.

Peppermint

One of the most popular essential oils, peppermint oil has a multitude of uses from treating a cold to sore muscles to relieving a stomach ache.

- **Energy** – Feeling tired in the middle of the day? Then, forget a caffeine shot and inhale the smell of peppermint oil—it will give you an instant lift. It is great for road trips and when studying. Add several drops to your shampoo for a pick me up in the morning.

- **Aid for Dieting** –If you feel hungry try inhaling peppermint oil to alleviate those hunger pangs. You can also place several drops of diluted oil on your collar bone or temples when you feel hungry to help relieve those food cravings.

- **Care of Muscles** – Add several drops of peppermint oil to a carrier oil such as sweet almond oil and rub directly on sore muscles to relieve pain and enhance healing.

- **Concentration and Focus** – It is claimed that smelling peppermint oil can help adults as well as children with ADHD gain added concentration and focus when undertaking tasks.

There are a multitude of ways to use peppermint oil, such as, to help with teething, colic and balancing hormones. As you learn more about the many uses of peppermint oil you will definitely want to keep this excellent essential oil in your health cabinet.

Chamomile

Chamomile possesses an inti-inflammatory calming action and is considered safe by both doctors and practitioners.

- **Calming** – Put several drops in some hot water, place a towel over your head and the bowl and inhale the steam.

- **Bruises, bites, stings, skin irritation** – Place several drops of chamomile in hot water and soak a cloth in the mixture to make a compress. Place the compress on the bruise. Alternatively, put several drops into a carrier oil and massage into the bruise. Use a similar procedure for bites, stings and skin irritation.

- **Allergies** – Place a diffuser in your home or office during the day and during allergy season to help lesson symptoms. You can also spray on your feet and inhale directly during serious flare-ups.

- **Irritability and Insomnia** – Inhale or drink chamomile tea to help experience the calming effects of this essential oil.

Chamomile is commonly used to fight infections, as an anti-inflammatory and as an anti-parasitic.

Eucalyptus

Eucalyptus is used as an analgesic and as an antibacterial, anti-inflammatory, insecticidal and expectant oil. It is mainly used in the respiratory system due to the fragrance of the oil as well as the way the scent affects people psychologically.

- **Increase Circulation and Blood Flow** – For circulatory system support. Put a drop into massage oil and rub into the skin to help increase circulation.

- **Improve Lung Function** – Whether it is asthma, bronchitis or congestion, lung function can be improved by using an inhalation tent to breathe in the steam.

- **Wakeup** – Whether you just feel tired when you wake up in the morning, or just have trouble waking up, or maybe you have jet lag, adding some diluted eucalyptus oil to your bath or shower can do wonders for your energy levels.

There are many other uses for eucalyptus oil, such as helping relieve the pain from kidney stones, or reducing pain generally. Eucalyptus is definitely one essential oil that you will want to keep handy around the home.

Lemon

Lemon essential oil is really versatile. It can be used as an antiseptic, in addition to its uses for cleansing and healing.

- **Concentration** – If you have a busy day ahead, then put a few drops of lemon oil into your skin lotion so that you can rub it on your arms and neck, inhaling deeply. You will be amazed at how your mind will be sharper and you will focus on your tasks better.

- **Alertness** – If you feel as if your day is dragging along and you feel a little lethargic, then try inhaling some lemon oil using a diffuser in the room you are working in.

- **Positivity** – Put several drops of lemon oil in candle wax (not on the flame), turn on some positive music and you will feel a real lift and less negative almost immediately.

- **Nausea** – Suffering from nausea due to morning sickness or as a side effect of medications you are taking? Then try putting several drops of lemon oil onto a cotton ball and sniff it each time you feel nauseous.

Lemon is so versatile and the smell is so clean and fresh that it is often added to shampoo, skin care and household cleaning products.

The above list is just a small selection of some of the most common essential oils that you can have in your basic care kit. There are many more. And as you knowledge and confidence grows, then you will want to experiment with many others. Studying what the various oils will do from a health standpoint will make a big difference to your wellbeing and quality of life.

You can use essential oils in so many different ways to improve and complement other methods of health care. Used correctly, you can accomplish a lot more than you ever thought possible.

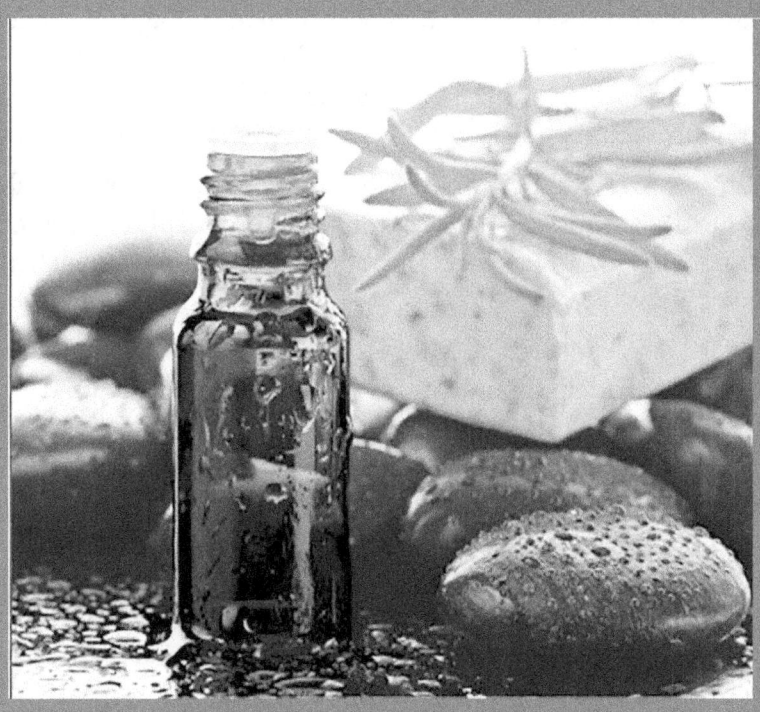

About The Author

Brian B Jacques started in business at a young age, and over the ensuing years, he has developed several very successful businesses. But his main interest for the past 35 years has been in natural health research and publishing.

Brian has presented seminars worldwide on such diverse subjects as Health Related issues, Motivation and Personal Development. In addition he has written numerous books, newsletters and articles on these subjects.

His very popular series of Mini Health Books has circulated widely around the world, and many more titles are in preparation.

Brian is a highly motivated individual, so much so that in 1985 he received a UK Industrial Society award for his work in the Motivation and Personal Development fields.

Brian has the following mottos:

- If something does not work out for you, then don't give up, but keep trying, trying, trying until finally you succeed.
- Success or failure in any endeavor is in your own hands.

Brian was born in the UK and lives with his wife in Florida, USA.

Index